Mode Deactivation Therapy
for Aggression & Oppositional
Behavior in Adolescents

An Integrative Methodology Using ACT, DBT & CBT

Jack A. Apsche, EdD, ABPP | Lucia R. DiMeo, PhD

New Harbinger Publications, Inc.

Publisher's Note

Distributed in Canada by Raincoast Books

Copyright © 2012 by Jack A. Apsche and Lucia R. DiMeo
New Harbinger Publications, Inc.
5674 Shattuck Avenue
Oakland, CA 94609
www.newharbinger.com

Acquired by Catharine Meyers; Edited by Stephen Brown; Cover design by Amy Shoup; Text design by Tracy Carlson; Index by James Minkin

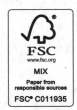

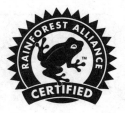

Library of Congress Cataloging-in-Publication Data

Apsche, Jack.
  Mode deactivation therapy for aggression and oppositional behavior in adolescents an integrative methodology using ACT, DBT, and CBT / Jack A. Apsche and Lucia R. DiMeo ; foreword by Robert J. Kohlenberg.
     p. cm.
  Includes bibliographical references and index.
  ISBN 978-1-60882-107-5 (pbk. : alk. paper) -- ISBN 978-1-60882-108-2 (pdf e-book) -- ISBN 978-1-60882-109-9 (epub)
  1. Adolescent psychotherapy. 2. Cognitive therapy for teenagers. 3. Aggressiveness in adolescence. I. DiMeo, Lucia R. II. Title.
  RJ503.A67 2012
  618.92'8914--dc23

                    2011050864

14 13 12

10 9 8 7 6 5 4 3 2 1   First printing

"For the clinician working with adolescents, mode deactivation therapy provides a practical and innovative approach to internalizing and externalizing disorders that takes concepts drawn from cognitive behavior therapy in new and interesting directions. The step-by-step approach to assessment and case conceptualization presented in this book is especially helpful and is the result of years of development work in the field."

—Steven C. Hayes, PhD, Foundation Professor of Psychology at the University of Nevada

"Working with angry, aggressive, and oppositional adolescents is fraught with significant challenges as well as rewards. This new guidebook should go a long way in diminishing the former while increasing the latter. The authors' empirically-supported therapy creatively integrates critical elements of other cognitive behavioral approaches into an easy-to-follow protocol that collaboratively engages adolescents in their own treatment."

—Robert Zettle, PhD, professor of psychology at Wichita State University and author of *ACT for Depression*

"For those of us who realize that medication alone is seldom effective for adolescents with aggressive and/or oppositional behaviors, *Mode Deactivation Therapy for Treating Aggression and Oppositional Behavior in Adolescents* is an essential companion. This therapeutic approach allies therapists with adolescents. Therapists learn to accept their clients in total and empower them to change. Jack Apsche and Lucia DiMeo have produced a book that is a must-read for any inpatient or outpatient clinician dedicated to understanding and treating the entire child—mind, body, and emotions."

—Robia A. Fields, MD, board-certified psychiatrist and medical director at a residential facility for children and adolescents

"Adolescents can be tough to treat under any circumstance. Sometimes, serious and complex psychological difficulties converge with that perfect storm of adolescent social development, individuation, and emotional upheaval, and the challenge is taken to a whole new level. Apsche and DeMio have done the hard work of integrating the best of evidence-based interventions and have created a tremendous resource targeting this extraordinarily challenging population."

—Kelly G. Wilson, PhD, associate professor at the University of Mississippi and author of *Mindfulness for Two* and *The Wisdom to Know the Difference*

Contents

Part I
Theory and Conception

Part II
The MDT Method from Assessment to Formulation

Part III
MDT in Action

Foreword

In my experience, the most challenging clinical work has been working with adolescents. This view has been echoed by many of my colleagues, which is why I am sure the work of Jack A. Apsche and Lucia R. DiMeo will be greatly appreciated by any clinician involved with treating adolescent clients. The theoretical and clinical insights offered in this book provide the clinician with an empirically supported and strategic methodology to help with some of the most difficult adolescent cases out there. The authors have done a remarkable job of developing a treatment protocol addressing comorbid psychiatric issues that can be used and implemented in a variety of therapeutic settings.

Mode Deactivation Therapy (MDT) was developed to target the complex typology of the adolescent population who experience comorbid Axis I disorders and concurrent Axis II thinking. When this thinking is evoked, it results in maladaptive and high-risk behaviors that impact the adolescent's ability to be successful at home, at school and in society.

MDT includes procedures for working with adolescents who have engaged in physical and sexual aggression, avoidance, oppositional behavior, fire setting, substance abuse and self-harm. One of the unique aspects of MDT is that the adolescent plays an active role in the therapeutic process. For instance, adolescents in MDT treatment are involved in building their own case conceptualization. As part of the process, they maintain an active role in connecting their beliefs to their behaviors, connecting their fears to what they avoid, and linking these relationships to their conscious and unconscious triggers. Since they are able to work collaboratively on this with their therapist, they tend to be more amenable to the process; thus, increasing rapport and trust with the therapist. As a result, some of the most difficult to treat adolescents become engaged in this process and maintain continued interest in participating in the treatment.

One of the most challenging aspects of treatment is facilitating the generalization of skills to life outside the therapist's office. Regardless of how many therapy sessions the adolescent is engaged in on a weekly basis, his/her progress is subject to end at the door to the office if the skills are not practiced and rehearsed during his/her time away from therapy. Mode Deactivation Therapy pays special attention to this problem. It is user friendly and lends itself to others learning and helping the adolescent practice these skills. For instance, in residential treatment facilities, this methodology is taught to the mental health staff working with the resident, and each staff member is trained to competency in the methodology. They learn to how to become aware of their resident's core beliefs and are able to use the well-defined Validate–Clarify–Redirect (VCR) intervention in order to help the youth obtain more productive beliefs. The method also includes instructions on how to use mindfulness interventions in psychoeducation groups and situational analyses in order to give the client an understanding of why he or she engaged in a particular behavior that resulted in a given consequence. Family therapy is also part and parcel of MDT, such that the home environment reinforces the MDT skills in the home. Incorporating the family as part of the MDT treatment occurs in residential treatment facilities, intensive outpatient programs, and routine outpatient settings. Families can be involved in developing a case conceptualization of their adolescent, assisting their child in engaging in mindfulness exercises and situational analysis, and understanding why their child may have acted out.

MDT is a treatment modality that provides an opportunity to understand why adolescents engage in the behaviors they do. MDT doesn't focus on helping clients relive their traumatic experiences; instead, it provides methods to help them understand and work on their beliefs that have developed from their life experiences. The method is aimed at helping clients see themselves and the world around them in a slightly different context and helping them change their behavior to make them more productive.

This book is a step-by-step guide to assist the clinician in understanding and implementing MDT with difficult adolescents. It is clearly written and walks the clinician through the entire treatment process from start to finish. Case examples and transcripts help the reader understand how to apply the methodology in session. The necessary tools such as the assessments are provided, and continuum scales can be applied to a variety of treatment settings as well.

Dr. Apsche and Dr. DiMeo have developed MDT over the last 10 years and this book distills the outcomes of empirical studies, trial and error through clinical application, and lessons learned over the years. Although in its early stages, the influence of MDT has already been observed to impact the lives of clients and their families. MDT has its origins in many treatment methodologies; however, its incorporation of evidence-based, third wave methodology has taken the approach to a new level of innovation. This book will be useful to clinicians treating some of the most complex and traumatized clients who enter their office. I fully expect that in the years to come, Dr. Apsche and Dr. DiMeo's book will have a significant role in adolescent therapy.

—Robert J. Kohlenberg, PhD, ABPP

Part I
Theory and Conception

Chapter 1

The Nature of
Adolescent Disorders

As an introduction to the nature of adolescent behavioral disorders, in this opening chapter we will briefly explore specific concepts of internalizing and externalizing dysfunctions and how they interact with particular adolescent conditions. However, these preliminary remarks are not meant to provide an exhaustive discussion on the topic, since other published works in the literature present detailed explanations and serve as valuable references in the understanding of adolescent behavioral intervention. Additionally, we expect that if you are reading this book as a clinician, you have already identified the pertinent symptomatology in your adolescent client. Therefore, we review a sampling of intervention programs currently available and briefly compare them to mode deactivation therapy (MDT). This provides (in our opinion) a more holistic perspective of adolescents with behavioral and emotional symptoms and lays the groundwork for the introduction of MDT—a treatment methodology that addresses the underlying interplay between internalizing and externalizing disorders in a specific and complex group of adolescents presenting anger, aggression, and oppositional behavioral issues.

We must also emphasize that this book is intended as an MDT treatment primer for adolescents with severe internalizing and externalizing disorders. For diagnostic purposes, we refer the reader to the *Diagnostic and Statistical Manual of Mental Disorders* (4th ed., text rev.; *DSM-IV-TR*; American Psychiatric Association, 2000). Furthermore, we believe that the MDT methodology presented in this book is relevant to all adolescents manifesting symptoms of opposition, anxiety, and trauma, with or without a formal mental disorder diagnosis. MDT is an evidence-based treatment for adolescents with comorbid Axis I disorders and concurrent Axis II beliefs that result in a variety of aberrant behaviors, including sexual aggression, physical aggression, anger, avoidance, fire setting, substance abuse and other forms of emotional and behavioral dysregulation. MDT's effectiveness in reducing internalizing disorders results in the de-escalation of the frequency and strength of the problem behaviors characteristic of externalizing disorders. A useful tool in the assessment of children and adolescents is Achenbach's (1991) Child Behavior Checklist (CBCL). This standardized instrument is distributed into three domains: internalizing disorders, externalizing disorders, and total score. The division of categories on the CBCL supports a major hypothesis of MDT; specifically, that it addresses the interplay of the internalizing disorder and Axis II beliefs to reduce the strength and frequency of the externalizing disorders.

We subscribe to Weisz and Kazdin's (2010) general grouping of internalizing and externalizing behaviors and disorders. From their perspective, and for the purpose of this book, internalizing disorders include anxiety, obsessive-compulsive disorders, depression, and trauma; while externalizing disorders include antisocial behaviors, disruptive behaviors, conduct disorders, anger and aggression, and attention deficit/hyperactivity disorder. Axis II beliefs are a derivative of Axis II disorders and were originally translated into beliefs by Beck, Freeman, and Associates (1990). They include beliefs associated with borderline, antisocial, avoidant, and dependent traits. Axis II beliefs are identified in MDT through the Compound Core Belief Questionnaire – S (CCBQ-S), presented in chapter 6 of this book. Externalizing and internalizing disorders, with or without Axis II beliefs, often combine in the adolescent as a complex typology that must be examined carefully in order to be treated successfully.

Kramer and Zimmermann (2009) hypothesized that fear and anxiety are at the core of adolescent internalizing and externalizing disorders, as well as aberrant behaviors. In other words, externalizing behaviors, such as physical aggression and excessive anger, are triggered by underlying fear and anxiety. MDT offers a clear path to identify these fear-based anxieties through the series of MDT assessments known as the Fear Assessments (introduced in chapter 5), which allow the clinician to determine the functional alternative of the fear, or the *avoids*. The avoids, or avoidance, identifies the phenomenon that Hayes (2004) refers to as experiential avoidance. We discuss this in more detail in chapter 7.

The variety of treatment methodologies and programs currently in use are a testament to the insidious effects of maladaptive adolescent behaviors. These behaviors have internal and external repercussions, as they are harmful to both the adolescent and those around the juvenile. We acknowledge the efficacy of many of the existing programs and recognize that MDT may even share similar approaches and techniques with them; however, we observe that the complex typology of the adolescent population is addressed more holistically and comprehensively with MDT. We find this to be true because MDT offers an extensive case conceptualization that determines the internalizing function of each problem behavior that the adolescent presents.

Internalizing Disorders

As previously mentioned, internalizing disorders include anxiety, depression, obsessive-compulsive disorder, and trauma, manifested by internalized behaviors, such as worry, sadness, or rumination. However, in adolescents, these disorders are also often expressed through a variety of aberrant externalized behaviors, for example, aggressiveness, opposition, or isolation from others.

Kendall, Furr, and Podell (2010) indicated that the prevalence rates for anxiety in the general adolescent population and primary core setting are around 10 to 20 percent. Cartwright-Hatton, McNicol, and Doubleday (2006) also reported that 3 to 24 percent have anxiety disorders. In a sample of 573 male adolescents with opposition and conduct disorders, Apsche, Bass, and DiMeo (2010) found that 53 percent presented some form of anxiety as measured by the MDT Fear Assessments. Kendall et al.'s data on children ages 7 to 13 suggested anxiety exists comorbidly as a tripartite construct that involves psychological, cognitive, and behavioral components. Accordingly, anxiety permeates the child's emotions, thoughts, and actions. As a result, the cognitive behavioral methodology developed by Kendall et al., "coping cat," is designed to address the internalizing disorders of anxiety in order to reduce its comorbidity with externalizing behavioral disorders in children and young adolescents. MDT expands the treatment of internalizing problems to reduce the strength and frequency of externalizing behaviors to include adolescents with severe conduct problems.

Depression in adolescents is a disorder with lethal, comorbid behaviors associated with suicide and parasuicide. Sadly, its prevalence continues to escalate. In 1996, Birmaher et al. reported that depression was present in 3 to 5 percent of the general adolescent population and in nearly 20 percent of adolescents by age 18. The National Institute of Mental Health (NIMH) identified suicide as the third leading cause of death in 2007 for young people ages 15 to 24. In 2003, Links, Gould, and Ratnayake reported on the prevalence of attempted and lethal suicide in adolescents and suggested that depression, existing comorbidly with a personality disorder, increases the likelihood of a lethal suicide. Apsche and DiMeo (2010) indicated that up to 20 percent of adolescents had symptoms of depression comorbid with anxiety, trauma, and personality beliefs. The complexities of depression comorbidity with other internalizing disorders as well as externalizing disorders, create a difficult therapeutic problem for clinicians in outpatient or clinical practice. Nonetheless, evidence-based treatments for depression have reported success for specific and well-defined populations of children and adolescents. Stark, Streusand, Krumholz, and Patel (2010) designed the ACTION treatment program for girls ages 9 to 13. The program is based on training in coping skills, problem solving related to emotional and stress issues, and recognition and reconstruction of cognitive core beliefs about self-worth. There are also cognitive behavioral therapy (CBT) group programs (Clarke & DeBar, 2010), as well as individual CBT programs for depression (Weersing & Brent, 2010) that are effective for specific populations of adolescents coping with depression.

Rohde, Clarke, Mace, Jorgensen, and Seeley (2004) conducted a randomized trial of Adolescents Coping with Depression (CWDA), a CBT program for depressed males 12 to 17 years old, and found that these youths had lower levels of aggressive and depressive symptoms after 12 months of treatment. However, reduction of symptoms of conduct disorder did not last or generalize past 12 months. Nonetheless, the potential for CWDA as a methodology that reduces both internalizing and externalizing disorders remains promising. There are numerous components of this program, including programmed muscular relaxation, that have a similarity to the mindfulness and imagery parts of MDT. Somewhat like CWDA, the Pittsburgh CBT program based on the work of Brent et al. (1997) offers an evidence-based methodology for depression and suicide in adolescents. The

Pittsburgh CBT program addresses negative thoughts about events related to apathy and helplessness through problem-solving and hypothesis-testing skills. Brent et al. suggested that this methodology might be effective for adolescents presenting depression, dysthymic disorder, and suicidality when applied outside of clinical trials in more real-world clinical care. CWDA targets the internalizing disorder of depression in order to reduce the behavior of apathy, agitation, and suicidality. In a systematic review of the effectiveness of interventions to reduce harm, Wethington et al. (2008) clearly made a case for the relationship between depression as an internalizing disorder and suicidality as an externalizing disorder. The basic principle of MDT theory is similar to this correlation: the behaviors associated with oppositional conduct, such as aggression and sexual abuse, are related to internalizing disorders left untreated.

According to Cohen, Mannarino, and Deblinger (2010), trauma-focused cognitive behavioral therapy (TF-CBT) addresses specific problems for children and adolescents between 3 to 18 years of age who have either witnessed or experienced trauma. Cohen et al. suggested that TF-CBT is an effective treatment for the multiple symptoms and disorders that children may experience following trauma. These symptoms may include depression and anxiety accompanied by behavioral, affective, cognitive, and psychological symptoms. TF-CBT is a hybrid form of CBT that incorporates several modalities of therapy into one, such as humanistic, attachment, and psychodynamic, as well as psychophysiology of childhood trauma (Cohen et al., 2010). However, although effective for the prescribed population of children and adolescents, TF-CBT is not intended to treat youth with conduct symptoms or who have been previously abused and are presenting symptoms of post-traumatic stress disorder (PTSD). MDT targets adolescents with conduct disorder characteristics, previous trauma, and Axis II beliefs and behaviors. TF-CBT does, however, follow the suggested MDT paradigm of addressing the internalizing disorder to reduce the strength and frequency of the externalizing disorder.

Externalizing Disorders

Externalizing disorders are conceived as disorders that are manifested in a variety of aberrant behaviors. These behaviors can include sexual and physical aggression, verbal aggression, suicidal and parasuicidal acts, substance abuse, and sometimes even criminal activity. Adolescents presenting these insidious behaviors are often frustrating for the clinician to treat due to the provocative nature of their opposition and resistance to life in general. Many of these behaviors fit the diagnostic category of the *DSM-IV-TR* (2000) referenced here for conduct disorder and oppositional defiant disorder. Unfortunately, many evidence-based treatments for these externalizing disorders are specifically designed for younger children; for example, Parent Management Training (Kazdin, 2005), Parent Management Training/Oregon Model (Forgatch & Patterson, 2010; Patterson, 1982), Anger Control Training (Lochman & Wells, 2004; Lochman, Wells, & Lenhart, 2008). Although effective, these approaches are meant for children ages 8 to 13, leaving out the older and more complex behaviorally and emotionally disturbed set of adolescents. Oregon's Multidimensional Treatment Foster Care (Chamberlain, 2003) was developed in an attempt to examine and test community-based alternatives to residential and long-term care facilities. It is a social learning-based modality with two primary goals: (1) to create opportunities for youths to live successfully in the community, and (2) to reunify them with their biological families. The treatment design appears effective and promising, yet it only focuses on the externalizing behaviors.

Multisystemic therapy (MST) is a widely published methodology with numerous randomized traits (Henggeler, 1982; Henggeler, Schoenwald, Borduin, Rowland, & Cunningham, 2009). More than 20 groups of independent reviewers support the effectiveness of MST in treating seriously delinquent and antisocial adolescents. Henggeler and Schaeffer (2010) indicated that MST encompasses strategies from several empirically supported theories, including, but not limited to: CBT, behavioral family therapy, motivational interviewing (MI), and behavioral parent training. MST suggests that cognitive behavioral therapy with the adolescent or together with family MST services (e.g., parent training, financial management, drug and alcohol services) is an effective treatment for substance abuse, sexual offending, and serious emotional disturbances (Henggeler & Schaeffer, 2010). Henggeler, Letourneau, et al. (2009) identified parental supervision and not engaging in deviant peer groups as the specific moderators of positive change in youth. The focus of MST appears to address the assumption that adolescent antisocial behaviors are a result of the interplay or risk factors embedded in the youth (Henggeler, Letorneau, et al., 2009) and suggests that mediating the externalizing systems results in positive outcomes for the adolescent and his or her family.

Greene and Ablon (2006) developed collaborative problem solving (CPS) for explosive children ages 6 to 12. The basis of their treatment model is to train the parent(s) and child to find a collaborative solution to problems, in order to reduce the child's aggressive behavior. Greene and Ablon believed that children's difficulties are not due to opposition or lack of motivation; instead their difficulties are based in cognitive deficits. CPS is hypothesized to mediate these cognitive deficits and reduce severe aggression. Although a great part of CPS methodology might be applicable to narrowly selected adolescent samples, the assumption that an adolescent is motivated, yet held back by cognitive deficits, may not be true in some cases. Many adolescents with conduct or oppositional defiant disorders are not motivated for treatment, as demonstrated by the results of MDT assessments (Apsche, 2010).

Summary

As we have indicated throughout this chapter, there are a number of valuable therapeutic modalities for children and adolescents. However, they often address a younger client population or have a limited symptomatology. As a result, these interventions may not comprehensively target the complex presentation of internalizing and externalizing behaviors in adolescents with severe anger, aggression, and oppositional behavior issues. That is when MDT is most effective. MDT treats adolescents with comorbid Axis I disorders (e.g., anxiety, depression, PTSD) and concurrent Axis II beliefs that result in a variety of behaviors including sexual aggression, physical aggression, avoidance, fire setting, and other forms of behavioral and emotional dysregulation. MDT is effective in reducing the internalizing disorders, which in turn decreases the frequency and strength of aberrant behaviors in externalizing disorders. The next chapter will provide an overview of the theoretical constructs of MDT and continue to develop the blueprint for MDT treatment.

Chapter 2

Theoretical Constructs of MDT and Literature Review

Mode deactivation therapy (MDT), at its core, is based on Beck's (1996) theoretical constructs of modes. Beck established that modes are composed of cognitive, affective, motivational, and behavioral elements that are integrated into an individual's personality and are activated during times of stress (1996, p. 2). In the case of adolescents, then, a mode generates psychological, physiological, and behavioral responses to events and thoughts. And, in fact, a mode represents the culmination of all of the adolescent's experiences and cognitions.

Modes are determined by *core beliefs* (schemas) that serve as the framework guiding the individual's thoughts, moods, and behaviors when responding to situations (Beck, Emery, & Greenberg, 1985). These core beliefs are both conscious and unconscious, acting as protective factors for the youth in adverse situations. Therefore, as a result of their reactivity to individual core beliefs, modes become a consistent and coordinated self-protective system for the adolescent. For example, an adolescent's perception of fear and danger can activate the system of modes as a form of protection and survival, as in the fear and flight response, or more typical of the kind of adolescents MDT treats—the fear and *fight* response.

The concept of modes and their relation to survival was further explained by Alford and Beck (1997) in their discussion on how modes and personality are rooted in the coordination of complex systems selected by the individual to ensure biological survival. It appears that these mechanisms of survival are always in a hypervigilant state and need only a catalyst—a precipitating event or perception—to begin a chain reaction. For example, a major problem in anxiety disorders is the activation of hypervigilant threat core beliefs or schemas that present in the individual as an exaggerated or faulty perspective of reality, and self-perception of a weak, helpless, and vulnerable person (Beck et al., 1985; Clark & Beck, 2010). This process can be explained as follows: The overevaluation of the perception of a threat activates the primal or instinctive threat mode in the individual, which, in turn, detects damage and seeks safety. When activated, this primal mode becomes even more hypervigilant and dominant, causing the internal threat appraisal to become overactivated, resulting in cognitive impairment; that is, distorting the individual's ability to adequately process the level of danger. In angry, aggressive, and oppositional adolescents, this may result in an exaggerated fear response and/or the perception of fear where none is evident, as well as the misinterpretation of the intentions and behaviors of others.

In other words, the primal or instinctive mode is the threat or fear reaction that surfaces in the adolescent to address basic survival or safety issues. This process can increase the perception of threat, simultaneously heightening the youth's sense of vulnerability and helplessness, while generating thoughts, images, and beliefs of danger (Clark & Beck, 2010). These cognitive vulnerabilities, as Clark and Beck refer to them, develop from negative childhood events such as trauma, neglect, humiliation, and abandonment. Moreover, they are associated with the concurrent activation of severe anxiety, as well as often thought to correlate to a potentially life-threatening or perceived life-threatening event.

Beck (1996) suggested that modes are prevalent in several clinical conditions or personality disorders, characterized by the presence of clusters of related dysfunctional beliefs that control information processing, interpretation, and memories in the individual. In other words, in the emotionally and behaviorally disordered adolescent, perceptions are skewed by the coupling of past experiences and by an activated mode. As a result, when an adolescent reacts (via mode activation) based on misinformation and distorted perceptions, a variety of aberrant behaviors occur.

Oppositional and conduct disordered adolescents remain in various levels of continuous hyperalertness and are extremely sensitive to mode activation when they perceive danger (real or not) or experience fear; thus, they are easily "charged," moving from a quiescent state into a highly activated state without notice (Barlow, 2002; Chorpita & Barlow, 1998; Clark & Beck, 2010). In MDT, understanding the mode activation process sets the groundwork for the effective therapeutic treatment of adolescents. MDT addresses cognitive vulnerabilities in the adolescent by helping the youth develop awareness of the connection between conscious or unconscious fears and mode system activation. The hypersensitive mode activation process explains the incidence of emotional dysregulation and impulse control issues in these youths (Apsche & Ward, 2003).

The Role of Childhood Trauma in Adolescents

As discussed above, a cognitive vulnerability for anxiety can develop in the adolescent through childhood experiences of trauma, abandonment, neglect, emotional invalidation, and/or humiliation. Emotional invalidation occurs when parents or caregivers are not warm or reinforcing and most likely are emotionally unstable. Clark and Beck (2010) reported that certain parenting practices such as "overprotection, restriction of individualization and autonomy and a preoccupation with potential danger and encouraging escape and avoidance" (p. 112), in response to perceived dangers or to anxiety, appear to significantly contribute to the cognitive vulnerability toward anxiety in adolescents (McNally, Malcarne, & Hansdottir, 2001). Johnson, Cohen, Brown, Smailes, and Bernstein (1999) made a correlation between sexual, physical, and emotional abuse and the development of personality and conduct disorders in adolescents. Childhood neglect was also linked to personality disorder symptoms in adolescents (Johnson et al., 2001; Johnson, Smailes, Cohen, Brown, & Bernstein, 2000). Furthermore, a history of abuse can be a precursor of post-traumatic stress disorder (PTSD), anxiety, and depression in adolescents. The abuse may also set the stage for the development of mixed personality traits, including clusters B and C markers (Apsche, Bass, Jennings, Murphy et al., 2005; Apsche, Bass, & Murphy, 2004). Cluster B includes antisocial, borderline, histrionic, and narcissistic traits, whereas Cluster C contains avoidant, dependent, and obsessive-compulsive traits (APA, 2000).

We have found that maladaptive core beliefs ingrained in personality traits and/or disorders often interfere with therapeutic success in the treatment of adolescents. Therefore, identifying the adolescent's conglomerate of beliefs before treating the anger, opposition, or aggression is critical to MDT, as explained in chapter 8. Additionally, because beliefs originate from different clusters and integrate with each other in their presentation, they serve the adolescent as a protective factor from abuse issues, while simultaneously making treatment more complex, and may in fact interfere with treatment. Consequently, not addressing these beliefs clinically becomes treatment-interfering behavior by the clinician.

Reactive and Proactive Aggression in Adolescents

Brown, Atkins, Osbourne, and Milnamow (1996) defined proactive aggression as an unprovoked aversive behavior intended to cause harm, overpower, or otherwise coerce another person, whereas reactive aggression is considered to be a defensive response to a perceived threat, fear, or provocation. In other words, proactive adolescents seek and gain benefits and rewards from aggressive acts, while reactive adolescents are guided by their emotional reactions or dysregulation in their aggression (Dodge, Lochman, Harnish, Bates, & Pettit, 1997). These views on aggression have theoretical roots in the frustration-aggression model posited by Dollard, Doob, Miller, Mowrer, and Sears (1939), later revisited and advanced by Berkowitz (1990). Although there are different correlates to proactive and reactive aggression, Dodge and Coie (1987) suggested that, nonetheless, they are statistically related. The understanding of the differences and commonalities of these two subtypes of aggression is important in treating adolescents with severe behavioral problems, since as many as 40 percent of reactive adolescents have traits of personality disorders (Dodge et al., 1997). These angry adolescents also often present self-punitive and self-critical characteristics and have a tendency to experience emotional numbness. Apsche and DiMeo (2010) indicated that reactive aggressive adolescents experience a higher incidence of emotional dysregulation, causing a distortion in their perceptions, which can result in aberrant responses.

A psychological profile of reactive adolescents includes a higher incidence of symptoms of depression, sleep disorders, somatization, and oppositional behavior, in addition to verbal and physical aggression (Dodge et al., 1997). A social history profile often reveals a prevalence of early trauma, including parental rejection, exposure to family violence, and family instability. Dodge et al. likened the behavior of reactive adolescents to that of individuals with borderline personality disorder in the shared tendency to interpret hostility in the communication of peers, as well as engage in dialectical thinking. However, they also proposed that dichotomous conflict (the struggle between control and impulsivity often found in reactively aggressive youth) and attention-seeking behaviors of these adolescents may be the precursors to actions that are sometimes interpreted by others as impulsive. Also of importance is the correlation between emotional dysregulation, aggression, and suicidal threats and gestures in adolescents (Koenigsberg et al., 2001). Furthermore, Dodge et al. indicated that angry, aggressive, and oppositional youth have a diminished ability in encoding relevant social cues, often as a result of misguided perceptions.

Apsche (2010) developed a 20-question scale to determine the adolescent's predominant score of reactive or proactive aggression. It appears that many adolescents have a "foot" in each category, suggesting that there might be a continuum of aggression that runs from reactive to proactive. This Reactive-Proactive Scale (included in chapter 4) goes from 1 to 10, with 1 being most reactive and 10 being most proactive. This continuum suggests that reactive aggression left untreated might become more proactive over time. The possible etiology of proactive and reactive aggression, which we believe is rooted in early childhood experiences, is significant to treatment.

The Development of MDT

The development of MDT dates back to the late 1990s when Jack Apsche, one of this book's coauthors, encountered frustration in the application of cognitive behavioral therapy (CBT) and social skills training (SST) in the treatment of male juvenile sex offenders presenting personality disorders and beliefs, severe disruptive behavior, and other psychiatric conditions. The efficacy of CBT and SST on this population proved limited, thereby providing the impetus for MDT's origin and development. Over a decade later, MDT has become an evidence-based methodology firmly grounded and effective in the treatment of behaviorally and emotionally disordered youth between the ages of 14 and 18. Most recently, MDT treatment has been extended to female adolescents and family systems. The next section will provide some documented highlights of MDT over the past 10 years. But first, a brief review of the four theories that influenced its development.

As mentioned at the beginning of this chapter, MDT is primarily based on Beck's (1996) theory of modes and on cognitive behavioral therapy. However, it also integrates elements from dialectical behavior therapy (DBT), functional analytic psychotherapy (FAP), and acceptance and commitment therapy (ACT). MDT incorporates DBT's "grain of truth" and "validating" a client's beliefs approach (Linehan, 1993; Linehan, Davidson, Lynch, & Sanderson, 2005), as well as explores "life and treatment interfering behavior," resulting in a therapeutic modality that doesn't challenge cognitive distortions but instead addresses life-interfering and treatment-interfering fears and beliefs in a collaborative manner. MDT adapts FAP's concept of "contingencies of reinforcement" (Kohlenberg

& Tsai, 1993) experienced in past relationships in order to target behavioral change cognitively and experientially during the therapeutic session, as well as in the client's daily life. Finally, MDT interweaves ACT's elements of "acceptance and defusion" (Hayes, Strosahl, & Wilson, 1999) together with mindfulness to emerge as MDT's *validation, clarification, and redirection* (VCR) components. The strength of MDT methodology lies in its ability to accept the adolescent where he or she is in the moment and to work in collaboration toward the creation of functional beliefs and behavior change. MDT empowers the youth to gain emotional and behavioral self-awareness and self-regulation. These tools become transferable skills to the individual's various endeavors throughout life and are instrumental in the reduction of aggression, self-harm, and oppositional behavior.

Mode Deactivation Therapy Pulls It All Together

Early in the development of MDT, it became evident that certain therapeutic factors provided a critical structure to the methodology. Some of these MDT elements are as follows:

- Treatment is goal oriented.

- Treatment is focused on beliefs.

- Each session is structured.

- The number of sessions is limited.

- The goals of therapy are clear.

- There is collaboration between therapist and client.

- The therapeutic relationship is measured.

- Treatment addresses resistance in client.

- Treatment empowers the client to become his/her own therapist.

- There are no cognitive distortions.

- A complete case conceptualization guides treatment.

- Treatment addresses modes.

- It is a mindfulness-based treatment.

- Acceptance of self and circumstances is integral to treatment.

- Emotional defusion is integral to treatment.

- Cognitive defusion is integral to treatment.

- Treatment addresses both didactic and experiential learning.

- Validation, clarification, and redirection address both cognitive and experiential learning.

- The functional alternative belief creates the possibility of change both cognitively and experientially.

- Fear is conceptualized as leading to avoidance.

- Treatment is for adolescents.

A comparison of therapeutic factors found in MDT, CBT, DBT, FAP, and ACT (see table 1 below) provides a clear map of the similarities and differences between MDT and its four influential treatment methodologies (Apsche, 2010).

Table 1. Comparison of MDT and Other Treatments*

Therapeutic Factors	MDT (Apsche & Ward, 2003)	CBT (Beck et al., 1990)	DBT (Linehan, 1993)	FAP (Kohlenberg & Tsai, 1993)	ACT (Hayes et al., 1999)
Goal-oriented treatment	Yes	Yes	Yes	Yes	Yes
Focus of treatment	Present, in-vivo work in sessions	Initially present focused	Present	Present	Present
Session structure	Yes, but flexible	Yes	Yes	Yes	Yes, but flexible
Session limitation	Yes, but flexible	Aims to be time-limited	Aims to be time-limited	Yes, but flexible	Yes, but flexible
Cognition	Unconscious & conscious	Conscious	Conscious	Conscious	Conscious
Goals for therapy	Yes: Empower patient to modify underlying beliefs to thereby change moods and behaviors (deactivate modes)	Yes: Uses variety of techniques to change thinking, moods, and behaviors	Yes: Skills training to better manage symptoms	Yes: Uses within-session contingencies to change behavior	Yes, but flexible

Collaboration between therapist and client	Yes	Yes	No	Yes	Yes
Therapeutic alliance important	Yes	Yes	Yes	Yes	Yes
Addresses resistance	Yes	No: Assumes patients will comply with treatment	Yes	Yes	Yes
Empowers client to be own therapist	Yes	Yes	No	No	Yes
Thoughts/ beliefs as dysfunctional	No: Beliefs are not thought of as dysfunctional, which invalidates the patient's experience. Beliefs are validated as being created out of a patient's experience, then are balanced to deactivate modes	Yes: Teach patient to identify, evaluate, and respond to their dysfunctional thoughts and beliefs with schema assumptions (scanning)	Yes: Balance through change and acceptance	Yes	No
Cognitive distortions	No: Thoughts/ beliefs are not distortions since they are based on past experience	Yes	No	Yes	No
Dialectical thinking	Yes: Focus on balancing	No	Yes: Focus on the dialectical pattern/process	No	Yes
Case conceptualization	Yes: Ever-evolving and drives treatment	Yes: Ever-evolving formulation of the patient's problems in cognitive terms	Yes: Important	Yes: Case formulation	Not specific

Case conceptualization is specific, typology driven	Yes	No	No	No	No
Change experiential learning through recreating positive experience	Yes	No	No	No	No
Acceptance and validation in the moment	Yes	No	Yes	No	Yes
Modes	Yes: Perceptions trigger physiological cues, which trigger beliefs (entire process is mode activating)	No	No	No	No
Triggers important	Yes: Learning the triggers is key to preventing activation of modes	Yes	No	N/A	No
Client's perceptions important	Yes: Perceptions trigger modes	No: Perceptions are distorted	Yes	Yes: Perceptions are based on past experiences	No
Reducing anxiety, addressing trauma	Yes: Uses exposure to fear cue to decrease perception of fear	No: Focuses on thought-feeling-behavior connection	No	No	No
Fear → avoids paradigm	Yes	No	No	No	No
Clear direct structured sessions for adolescents	Yes	No: Cognitive distortion based	No: Uses esoteric skill training	No	Metaphors only
Evidence-based for adolescents only	Yes	No	No	No	No

*Adapted from *Mode Deactivation Therapy: The Complete Guidebook for Clinicians* (Apsche, 2010).

MDT systematically assesses and restructures dysfunctional *compound core beliefs* (schemas) into *functional alternative beliefs* in the adolescent (Apsche, Ward Bailey, & Evile, 2003). In MDT, core beliefs are acknowledged and validated as legitimate truths for the adolescent—no matter how irrational. They are perceived as a result of past experiences and represent the "grain of truth" for the adolescent at a particular time. MDT collaborates with the adolescent to balance and deactivate maladaptive mode responses and transform them into functional beliefs. The validation, clarification, and redirection (VCR) process in MDT is used to balance beliefs and regulate emotions. Validation promotes unconditional acceptance of conscious and unconscious experiences. Clarification provides an alternative perspective of the past experiences and present circumstances. Redirection measures the possible acceptance of a slightly different belief. Through MDT, adolescents learn that there is a perceptual continuum instead of an "all or nothing" state. The movement from dichotomous and dialectical thinking redirects and provides the adolescent with a new awareness, resulting in opportunities for alternative behavior. Finding the grain of truth in the adolescent's perception is at the core of MDT. It serves as the basis for the treatment of personality beliefs and traits that result in aggression and misinterpretation of events. MDT employs a number of assessments and continuums that evaluate the adolescent's level of truth, trust, fear, and belief. These measures serve both the client and the clinician as a barometer of the youth's perceived reality and rationale for behavior.

To reiterate, MDT's stance is that the adolescent's concept of reality and perception is shaped by past experiences. Therefore, in therapy, present behavior is evaluated in the context of reinforcement history. Acceptance, mindfulness, and defusion techniques have been adapted into MDT to teach adolescents awareness and healthy alternatives to thoughts, feelings, memories, and physical sensations that in the past have caused fear and emotional dysregulation. In a nutshell, MDT is the following:

- An extensive case conceptualization

- Mindfulness

- Acceptance

- Defusion

- Validation, clarification, and redirection of functional alternative beliefs

Evidence of MDT's Effectiveness

After over 10 years of MDT's use in the therapeutic setting, there is ample evidence of the significant reduction of severe behavioral symptomatology after individual or family MDT treatment. For example, one of the first documented case studies of the clinical application of MDT (Apsche & Ward,

2003) revealed a marked reduction in physical and verbal aggression in an adolescent previously unsuccessful in treatment. An additional benefit of treatment was a decrease in the youth's anxieties and fears. Because anxiety and fear can serve as mode activators and instigate a chain reaction of cognitive and behavioral dysfunction in the adolescent, they are critical targets in MDT treatment.

Sexual offending behavior, including physical and sexual aggression, was significantly reduced through MDT compared to CBT or SST (Apsche, Bass, Jennings, Murphy, et al., 2005; Apsche et al., 2004; Apsche, Bass, Siv, & Matteson, 2005; Apsche & Ward, 2003). This is in part a result of how MDT treatment addresses both internal behaviors (e.g., anxiety and depression) and external behaviors (e.g., aggression) in adolescents. MDT also significantly reduces maladaptive behaviors and psychological distress associated with conduct and personality disorders compared to CBT (Apsche et al., 2004). Most importantly, a two-year posttreatment study conducted by Apsche, Bass, and Siv (2005) revealed significantly reduced recidivism rates for sexual offenses and severe aggressive behavior in male adolescents treated with MDT in residential settings, as compared with adolescents treated with CBT and SST, as illustrated in table 2.

Table 2. Recidivism Rates of Apsche, Bass, and Siv (2005) Study

Therapeutic Treatment	Recidivism Rate	Behavior
MDT	7%	No sexual offenses
CBT	20%	Includes sexual offenses and aggravated assault
SST	49.5%	Includes sexual offenses, murder, aggravated assault, auto theft, sale of controlled substances

Treatment comparison studies between MDT and CBT and SST have documented greater therapeutic success of MDT in the treatment of adolescents with the more complex typologies of severe behavioral difficulties. For example, as previously mentioned, MDT was initially applied to an adolescent male population of sex offenders. Within this population there was a prevalent comorbidity of Axes I and II diagnoses. The most common Axis I diagnoses included conduct disorder, oppositional defiant disorder, and post-traumatic stress disorder. Recurrent Axis II diagnoses included borderline personality traits, narcissistic personality traits, histrionic personality traits, dependent personality traits, avoidant personality traits, and mixed personality traits. Murphy and Siv (2007) conducted a replication study comparing the efficacy of MDT methodology to the current Treatment as Usual (TAU) for aggressive adolescent males in residential treatment. Results suggested greater reduction of symptoms of depression and suicidal ideation after the application of MDT.

The success of MDT in residential settings led to its implementation in outpatient settings. Apsche and Bass (2006) conducted an outpatient replication study of the 2005 MDT inpatient study of male adolescents with conduct disorder (Apsche, Bass, Jennings, & Siv, 2005). Results revealed a significant reduction in recidivism of such behaviors as aggressive and defiant behavior, school suspensions, and symptoms of psychological distress in adolescents diagnosed with conduct and personality disorders compared to TAU. MDT as an outpatient intervention is now being employed with both male and female adolescents.

Apsche, Bass, Zeiter, and Houston (2009) suggested that family MDT not only can be effective during treatment, but can generalize to the home environment. Apsche, Bass, Zeiter, et al. completed a family MDT clinical study of 14 adolescents who evidenced such problems as sexual and physical aggression, as well as oppositional behaviors including verbal aggression (Apsche & Bass, 2010). The results indicated that MDT outperformed TAU. At 18 months of observation, the MDT group had zero incidents of sexual recidivism, while the TAU group had 10 reported incidents. The MDT group reported 3 incidents of physical aggression while the TAU group reported 12. These results are favorable for MDT as a family therapy and indicate that further studies with larger groups would be beneficial (Apsche, Bass, & Siv, 2006). Additionally, outcome data suggest that MDT shows promise as an effective outpatient family treatment approach (Apsche, Bass, & Houston, 2007).

A meta-analysis of 38 MDT studies (published and unpublished) conducted by Apsche in 2009 included 458 male adolescents from individual studies, 61 from family MDT studies, and 30 from the replication study (Apsche & DiMeo, 2010). From the individual studies, 204 participants had conduct disorder and 254 had sexual offenses. Comorbidity of Axis I and Axis II diagnoses was prevalent among the sample population. Fifty-two percent were diagnosed with conduct disorder, 45 percent with oppositional defiant disorder, 51 percent with post-traumatic stress disorder, and 20 percent with other Axis I disorders. Axis II diagnoses included 58 percent with mixed traits, 40 percent with borderline personality traits, 2 percent with histrionic personality traits, 30 percent with dependent personality traits, and 20 percent with avoidant personality traits. A history of abuse was also present in the majority of the sample population for individual cases: 92 percent experienced four types of abuse (verbal, physical, sexual, and neglect), 54 percent witnessed violence, and 28 percent presented parasuicidal behaviors (Apsche & DiMeo, 2010, p. 298).

The meta-analysis data indicated the effectiveness of MDT with adolescent males ages 14 to 18. The effect size for the target behaviors, specifically, physical aggression for both the conduct groups and the sexual abusing groups, demonstrated a large effect size and Cohen's d. The sexual abusing group had a large effect size for their sexual behaviors while in treatment and for two years in post-treatment. MDT had a large effect size and Cohen's d effect in all areas of the Child Behavior Checklist (CBCL) and the State-Trait Anger Expression Inventory (STAXI). The CBCL and the STAXI indicated a reduction of anxiety and anger. The results of this assessment data support our hypothesis that MDT can reduce internalizing disorders in the adolescent, resulting in a de-escalation of aberrant behaviors associated with externalizing disorders. It is important to note that although MDT has in small samples reduced parasuicidal behavior; it has no effect on the reduction of symptoms as measured by the Beck Depression Inventory – 2 (BD-2) and the Suicide Ideation Questionnaire High School (SIQHS). Further studies of MDT may clarify, confirm, or disprove this hypothesis.

Summary

Although primarily derived from Beck's (1996) theory of modes and cognitive behavioral therapy (CBT), MDT also integrates elements from dialectical behavior therapy (DBT), functional analytic psychotherapy (FAP), and acceptance and commitment therapy (ACT). MDT targets angry, aggressive, and oppositional adolescents. It acknowledges and validates the adolescent's experiences and reality, promoting the exploration of the grain of truth and personality beliefs. Cognitive distortions are not challenged; rather they are discussed for the purpose of transforming them into functional beliefs. The clinician examines the adolescent's reinforcement history in order to better understand the presence of pervasive behaviors and fears. Acceptance, mindfulness, and defusion are practiced to teach the youth how to balance perceptions and interpretations of internal and external stimuli. MDT aims at changing and shaping behaviors in session and reinforcing their execution out of session. Overall, as a CBT methodology, MDT addresses the adolescent's specific internalizing disorder, which results in the remediation of the maladaptive behaviors of the externalizing disorders. Throughout this book, we present this methodology step-by-step.

Chapter 3

MDT as a Third Wave Treatment

Third wave behavior therapies look more at the function and context of individuals than at their structure. These therapies also emphasize experiential change strategies as well as didactic ones (Hayes, 2004). Many of the third wave methodologies use mindfulness and acceptance strategies to allow for the process of change. However, the goal of these therapies is not to do away with problems, thoughts, or emotions, but rather to learn to accept them for what they are—private internal experiences, not truths (O'Brien, Larson, & Murrell, 2008). Both ACT and MDT are considered third wave therapies. ACT, in fact, had a profound impact on one of the authors of this book (Jack Apsche) during his development of MDT, as we briefly highlight in this chapter.

MDT and ACT

ACT's influence is palpable throughout MDT. Nonetheless, MDT was developed separately from ACT and indeed, the early development of MDT focused largely on the use of assessments, case conceptualization, and validation strategies to treat mostly juvenile male sex offenders. My (J. Apsche) experiences in ACT workshops and readings propelled me to further evaluate this exciting new methodology. Although at the time, ACT seemed more homogeneous in its treatments, focusing mostly on such problems as anxiety and depression, its brilliant use of acceptance, functional contextualism, language, defusion, and mindfulness made me wonder whether these elements could be adapted to treat an angry, aggressive, and often deviant adolescent population. The answer was yes, with some adjustments. As a result, the ACT elements (or sometimes derivatives) mentioned above are evident throughout MDT methodology, but not always exactly as they may appear in ACT. Overall, MDT integrates some aspects of ACT, while maintaining its own identity and methodology in order to effectively address the treatment of adolescents with severe emotional and behavioral disorders. In the next section, we briefly highlight some of the relevant therapeutic factors, first as they present in ACT and then as they are incorporated into MDT.

Functional Contextualism and Case Conceptualization

Hayes et al. (1999) explained that ACT is based on a philosophy of science identified as *functional contextualism*. This concept requires the practitioner to analyze behaviors in terms of their specific function within a discrete context. MDT's exhaustive case conceptualization serves as the foundation of its own functional contextualism. In other words, through MDT case conceptualization, the function of the adolescent's internal and external fears, beliefs, and behaviors are identified and targeted for treatment. Chapters 7, 8, and 9 review MDT case conceptualization.

Language and Functional Alternative Beliefs

Greco and Hayes (2008) delineated how ACT goes beyond "abnormalities" and diagnosis and focuses on the contextual processes that are particularly concerned with language. ACT postulates that a great part of psychological suffering is generated by language processes that trap the individual and result in psychological inflexibility. MDT also follows these linguistic theoretical postulates and creates a pathway to psychological flexibility through the focus on functional alternative beliefs that are validated in the moment by the clinician, parent, and adolescent. The functional alternative belief is the opposite (to a degree) of the youth's dysfunctional or unhealthy beliefs. We discuss functional alternative beliefs in chapter 9.

Acceptance

Hayes (1994) identified acceptance as one of the most important contextual change strategies in an individual. In this manner, acceptance refers to the conscious abandonment of a direct change agenda in the key domains of private events, self, and history—and openness to experiencing thoughts and emotions as they are, not as the client says they are. Dougher (1994) asserted that the key component of acceptance is letting go of one's control agenda and orienting oneself toward valued actions. It appears then that acceptance is not a goal in and of itself, but is a method of empowering the achievement of life goals. MDT embraces acceptance as integral to its treatment modality, but moreover makes it relevant to the youth in treatment. We believe that acceptance is the ability to relate to and participate in difficult thoughts and emotions in the moment, as well as to accept that these painful emotions and thoughts will occur throughout one's lifetime. Chapter 10 further explores the concept of acceptance.

Experiential Avoidance

Hayes et al. (1999) viewed *experiential avoidance* as the opposite of acceptance. O'Brien et al. (2008) defined experiential avoidance as the situation that occurs when an individual is either unwilling or too fearful to remain in contact with painful emotions, situations, thoughts, or memories. Hayes, Wilson, Gifford, Follette, and Strosahl (1996) explained this process as a lack of acceptance of private events (an individual's thoughts) as they occur in an uncontrolled and an unregulated manner. MDT conceptualizes avoidance from a *fear* ➔ *avoids* paradigm in which the adolescent avoids what he or she fears. This schema is further explained in chapter 7.

Defusion

ACT refers to *defusion* as a weakening of the literal, evaluative function of language; that is, separating the "words" from the emotions. MDT looks at defusion as two separate events: *emotional defusion* and *cognitive defusion*. It targets emotions associated with avoidance-based cognitions through emotional defusion, the process that evolves from where the emotional pain is actually located in the body. Cognitive defusion helps the adolescent de-escalate (defuse) the effect of his or her emotionally laden thoughts. This is based on the hypothesis that the power of the adolescent's avoidance is based both in language and in emotion (fear). Therefore, defusing the power of language cognitions and emotions is part of the MDT methodology. The process of defusion allows the adolescent the opportunity to experience the thoughts and feelings that have created avoidance so that the youth can accept them as part of himself or herself. Chapter 10 delineates emotional and cognitive defusion.

Mindfulness

The practice of mindfulness permeates ACT treatment, from clinicians to clients. In *Acceptance and Mindfulness Treatments for Children and Adolescents: A Practitioner's Guide*, Greco and Hayes (2008) highlighted the efficacy of using mindfulness in treating adolescents. The authors claimed that individuals who voluntarily begin a mindfulness practice often have a "beginner's mind"—that is, they are open and ready to learn, enthusiastic, and not cynical. Unfortunately, adolescents who engage in MDT treatment are oftentimes oppositional and cynical. Nonetheless, MDT is grounded in a mindfulness-based methodology. We believe that mindfulness is to be fully present in the moment, without judgment. We also subscribe to the need for the clinician to have a personal mindfulness practice in order to be successful when treating youth with MDT. We have found that mindfulness concepts practiced by the clinician openly and honestly will positively transfer to even the angriest adolescent because they become "real." Although chapter 11 provides a number of mindfulness exercises, we want to begin to establish the context of mindfulness in MDT before you continue with the next chapters.

Preview to MDT Mindfulness

As mentioned above, the real practice of mindfulness by the MDT clinician becomes a great bridge to building an effective, collaborative relationship with the client. One easy way to begin is by teaching the adolescent breathing exercises. The youth is then joined in each breathing and mindfulness exercise by the clinician. These are simple exercises designed to build upon each other. Although they are presented in greater detail in chapter 11, we would like you to begin the experience of MDT mindfulness and awareness now. The following exercise is intended for both the clinician and the adolescent. We suggest that the clinician practice it prior to implementing it with the adolescent as a way to increase his or her understanding of mindfulness and make it "real" in MDT work. This basic exercise helps you become more aware of your thoughts, feelings, and even physical sensations. Developing self-awareness is the first step in becoming more aware and empathetic to others' feelings and emotions. The following exercise consists of three parts: awareness, description, and redirection. Make yourself comfortable, close your eyes, and let's begin:

1. Awareness

   Observe and notice your surroundings, thoughts, feelings, and different bodily sensations. Are you thinking about being on the beach right now? Do you feel relaxed as if you are at the beach? Or are you thinking about a peer who is giving you a hard time and feel tense? What you are thinking is affecting how you are feeling; therefore your physical body is reacting.

2. Describe

   Put your observations into words and say how you feel. You can start by saying what you see: describe to yourself the "scene" that you are seeing in your mind. What or whom are you thinking about? Does this "scene" make you feel positive or negative, anxious or excited? If you don't want to say it out loud, write it down!

3. Redirect Yourself

   Slowly redirect your attention to your breath. Follow your breath—in…and…out…
   Breathe in…count one…
   Expand yourself…
   Slowly…
   Expand your attention to your whole body…
   Try to sense any discomfort, tension, or resistance…
   Just feel whatever you feel…breathe in…breathe out…

Allow yourself to feel whatever you feel…
Become aware of your feelings…
You have experienced a piece of mindfulness and awareness.

(Apsche & DiMeo, 2010, pp. 288–289)

After completing this exercise and realerting yourself, notice your feelings and emotions. Do you feel more relaxed, calmer, and more alert? Sometimes, taking a moment to yourself, like in the previous exercise, can renew your energy and enthusiasm for life. Developing balance in your own life can assist you when working therapeutically with angry, aggressive, and oppositional adolescents. Additionally, a mindfulness practice facilitates the process of what we call in MDT *balancing beliefs* through validation, clarification, and redirection.

Validation, Clarification, and Redirection

The validation, clarification, and redirection (VCR) process is unique to mode deactivation therapy. MDT integrates mindfulness, acceptance, and defusion with validation, clarification, and redirection (VCR) of the functional alternative belief (FAB), or balanced beliefs. A functional alternative belief becomes a balanced belief the moment it is accepted by the adolescent to some degree, on a scale of 1 to 10. The purpose of the validation, clarification, and redirection process of the functional alternative belief is to reinforce the adolescent's experience both emotionally and cognitively. That is, it allows the youth to experience positive validation for his or her balanced belief. This process is discussed in chapters 9 and 10.

The Resistant Adolescent and Collaboration

Adolescents, especially oppositional adolescents, often do not want to be in therapy. Although parents, judges, or other "officials" may mandate treatment, the adolescent often thinks that he/she is fine. As a result, the therapeutic task is often challenging. However, for a clinician practicing MDT, the treatment process might prove less difficult. Let's explain how that might work. First, you begin MDT with mindfulness. You need not discuss "issues" or problems; instead you work with the youth to be present in the moment. This requires the MDT clinician to be there, joined with the client in awareness, because if you as a clinician do not practice mindfulness, neither will the adolescent. MDT mindfulness requires honest effort and, again, being real, in the moment. MDT also involves the completion of a series of specific assessments in order to develop the case conceptualization. Validation and collaboration are embedded throughout the assessment and case conceptualization process. As discussed in chapter 2, the Reactive-Proactive Scale measures the nature of the adolescent's aggression. We have found a positive correlation between high resistance and high proactive scores, which, in turn, seem to predict a higher incidence of denial of problems by the youth. The MDT assessments are effective with a variety of adolescents presenting behaviors ranging from cooperative to oppositional and negative. Although nothing prevents an adolescent from totally refusing to cooperate in the therapeutic environment, it happens rarely when implementing MDT. Interestingly, even the most defiant and oppositional adolescents appear responsive to the specific MDT assessments designated for him or her. This may be in part because the mindfulness and collaborative case conceptualization process systematically address resistance and opposition by validating and shaping responses. Nonetheless, in chapter 5 we provide some suggestions for working with adolescents reluctant to complete assessments.

Summary

MDT, as a third wave therapeutic methodology, is structured in a manner that provides an effective framework for adolescent treatment. Although it is a therapeutic framework, MDT treatment is never linear or "cookbook" in nature as you will see when you begin to incorporate other components of MDT presented throughout this book. There is a well-defined similarity in the use of mindfulness, acceptance, and defusion between ACT and MDT. However, MDT takes the cognitive defusion presented in ACT and adds emotional defusion to complete the process. MDT also continues to explore the use of mindfulness, breathing, and imagery as time in treatment progresses. It uses these mindfulness practices to develop trust and a collaborative alliance between clinician and adolescent. In chapter 4, we take you step-by-step through the MDT assessment process in preparation for case conceptualization. Take your time as you read through the book so that these concepts can become your blueprint to adolescent treatment.

Part II

The MDT Method from Assessment to Formulation

The MDT Assessments

This chapter presents general guidelines for administering MDT assessments. It also immerses you in the immediate use of instrumentation through the Beliefs about Therapeutic Alliance, the Typology Survey, and the Reactive-Proactive Scale. All assessments are provided in their entirety for your understanding and use. To further explain MDT's therapeutic approach to angry, aggressive, and oppositional adolescents, a distinction between a content, problem-based approach and a contextual framework is discussed.

Preparing for the Assessments

MDT is centered on a step-by-step, comprehensive assessment procedure culminating in a case conceptualization that guides treatment. To understand the methodology, it is important to engage in Socratic questioning. Never accept assumptions based on nonempirical hypotheses. Ask, "If so… then what"—continue to question throughout the MDT process. You are like a detective looking for clues, except that the clues relate to the internal core beliefs of the adolescent in treatment. The assessment process itself is both revealing and therapeutic. Therefore, it is important to prepare yourself, the youth, and the environment for optimal success. Take time to practice the administration, scoring, and interpretation of MDT instruments to develop your understanding and skills. Evaluate the physical environment where you meet with your adolescent—it is critical that the atmosphere be conducive to building rapport. Therefore, reduce distractions during assessments; a quiet setting will facilitate greater effectiveness. Additionally, consider the following suggestions before you administer an assessment: Conduct all assessments verbally, except the Beliefs about Therapeutic Alliance, presented in this chapter. In other words, do not just give the assessment to your client to complete; instead have the youth verbally discuss the questions with you, writing the responses on the protocol form (Apsche, 2010). Always explain the purpose of the assessment to the adolescent before initiating it. Here are some brief descriptions you can use: the Fear Assessment (chapter 5) examines the adolescent's relationship with trauma and experiential avoidance. The Compound Core Belief Questionnaire – S, or CCBQ-S (chapter 6), examines the youth's relationship to a variety of beliefs that often activate behaviors. Try to create a relaxed atmosphere in order to maintain good communication with the adolescent, taking breaks as needed throughout the procedure. In fact, some assessments may take more than one session to complete. You can make assessments relevant to the youth by using real-life examples, such as vignettes typical to adolescents or from your experiences in using the assessments. Finally, make sure that you are familiar and comfortable with the assessment before administering it, and approach each session in a collaborative manner.

MDT Therapeutic Alliance

A collaborative relationship between therapist and client is a cornerstone of MDT treatment. The clinician regularly monitors the therapeutic relationship through the Beliefs about Therapeutic Alliance. This 15-item assessment is completed separately by both the adolescent and the therapist at 30, 90, and 120 days into MDT treatment. Results are compared for agreement on 15 measures related to the youth's and clinician's perceptions. The adolescent responds as he/she perceives the relationship. The clinician responds as he/she perceives the youth could answer these measures. The items are scored individually, as well as per total score. The difference between the two scores (the clinician's and youth's) is the area of focus for both the therapist and the client. For example, if the response to the item "My therapist has my best interest at heart" by the adolescent is a 3 and the therapist's response is a 7, the difference of 4 points is an area of concern due to the large disparity between responses. This disparity suggests that the therapist and the youth are not in sync in their perceptions of one another. Therefore, the differences in the individual responses are of more concern than the actual individual value credited to the responses (Apsche, 2010). Take a look at the Beliefs about Therapeutic Alliance assessment presented next.

Beliefs about Therapeutic Alliance

Name: _____ Date: _____

Completed by Youth: _____ Therapist: _____

Listed below are some statements about your relationship with your therapist. Please read each statement and rate how much you agree or disagree.

	Totally Disagree	Disagree Very Much	Disagree Slightly	Neutral	Agree Slightly	Agree Very Much	Totally Agree
1. My therapist has my best interests at heart.	1	2	3	4	5	6	7
2. I (the youth) willingly participate in treatment.	1	2	3	4	5	6	7
3. I (the youth) actively participate in therapeutic assignments.	1	2	3	4	5	6	7
4. I (the youth) have confidence that my therapist can support me through difficult emotional times.	1	2	3	4	5	6	7
5. I (the youth) have demonstrated the ability to resolve conflicts.	1	2	3	4	5	6	7
6. I (the youth) understand that my therapist will tell me things I don't want to hear, for my own good.	1	2	3	4	5	6	7
7. I have confidence that my therapist will keep appointments with me as scheduled.	1	2	3	4	5	6	7
8. If my therapist makes a commitment to me, he/she will keep the commitment.	1	2	3	4	5	6	7
9. I have faith that no matter how bad my emotions feel, my therapist will understand me.	1	2	3	4	5	6	7

10. I am matched with a therapist who really is interested in my success in treatment.	1	2	3	4	5	6	7
11. I would pick my therapist to work with me if I were going to outpatient therapy.	1	2	3	4	5	6	7
12. I (the youth) often engage in behaviors to avoid my therapy sessions.	1	2	3	4	5	6	7
13. I (the youth) feel anxious and/or depressed prior to, following, or during a therapy session.	1	2	3	4	5	6	7
14. I know my therapist will be there to give the emotional support necessary.	1	2	3	4	5	6	7
15. I (the youth) accept some responsibility for problem behaviors when confronted within a reasonable period of time.	1	2	3	4	5	6	7

© 2009 Jack A. Apsche, EdD, ABPP

The clinician/youth collaboration continues through the completion of all MDT assessments (Typology Survey, Fear Assessments, and the Compound Core Belief Questionnaire – S), the Case Conceptualization, and the entirety of MDT treatment.

Content-, Problem-Based Approach vs. Contextual Framework

When beginning MDT with an adolescent, the level of rapport between the therapist and the youth at the time this new methodology is introduced will dictate the degree to which a "switch" in therapeutic focus is required, since the clinician may be moving from content to context, in which case the therapist shifts from a content-, problem-based approach to a contextual framework (Apsche, 2010). This reorganization is critical since in a problem-focused approach the treatment plan's goals and objectives, as well as clinical strategies, tend to focus on behaviors and on the content of life rather than on the context of change. For example, a treatment plan that is content-based may suggest:

Problem/Focus Area (1): Aggression

- *J. will identify past events in his life that led to his inability to remain in a community setting through developing a timeline with the help of his therapist over the next 30 days.*

While a treatment plan that is context-based may suggest:

Focus Area (1): Aggression

- *J. will begin to build a therapeutic relationship through increasing trust with his therapist and family in the next 30 days.*

- *In collaboration with his therapist, J. will gain an understanding and accept the relationship between aggressive behavior and adverse childhood experiences within the next 30 days.*

- *J. will identify triggers, fears, beliefs, and things that he avoids that result in aggressive behavior with the collaboration of his therapist within the next 30 days.*

This shift in clinical focus provides relief to the adolescent and promotes *clinical attractiveness*, which is enhanced through a form of *radical acceptance* (Apsche & Ward Bailey, 2003). Radical acceptance constitutes the adolescent's total acceptance of self, situation in life, past actions, history of abuse, and other experiences. Clinical attractiveness is increased through validating the adolescent's low levels of commitment to treatment and trust, thereby meeting the needs of the youth at the moment. This is very helpful in moving the youth into this shift in treatment and decreases the adolescent's perceived resistance (Tate, Reppucci, & Mulvey, 1995). By moving from the content of the youth's life to the context of the functional alternative belief (FAB); that is, the healthy or functional alternative belief to the core dysfunctional belief, you begin the shift toward change in the adolescent. Throughout this process, you collaborate with the youth to reach full acceptance of being who and where he or she is and allow the adolescent to accept and describe the fear, pain, and emptiness. This represents acceptance and defusion. Mindfulness exercises help guide this journey and are a part of the "awareness" of defusion.

The clinician can present radical acceptance to the youth by putting behavioral concerns in the proper context. Radical acceptance requires a reference to the target behaviors as typical responses to adverse life experiences. The goal is for the youth to understand past life experiences as causing overcompensating behaviors in situations that are perceived as threatening but may not actually have to be.

When shifting from a content-, problem-based focus to a context-based focus, it is important to develop trust of the new process with the youth. It may be helpful to keep in mind that your definition of trust may not be the same as the adolescent's. For example, the concept of trust to a clinician may mean confidence that no harm will come from interactions with another. On the other hand, a youth with issues of abuse or neglect may view trust as the ability to predict responses from someone or the potential to receive support from the other person, regardless of the situation. It is also important to create an atmosphere of trust and cooperation by clarifying beliefs that may cause the youth to distrust the process itself. This trust and cooperation is nurtured from the beginning; for example, as you complete the Typology Survey, give the adolescent a sense of control by encouraging honesty rather than embellishing or fabricating an answer when he or she isn't comfortable answering a particular question. You can always come back to the question later when more trust has been established. At all times, avoid an adversarial or one-up/down tactic with the youth (Apsche, 2010).

The Typology Survey

The Typology Survey provides detailed background information about the youth and is the basis for determining the type of Fear Assessment (chapter 5) to administer; additionally, it is critical for completing the Case Conceptualization (chapter 7). There are 12 sections to the Typology Survey, so it is important to familiarize yourself with its content and process before meeting with the adolescent, as well as consult with parents or caregivers for additional information.

The adolescent should be given an opportunity to consent to the assessment. So, inform the youth of the process that will take place during the session. Tell him/her the nature of the assessment and its purpose, and enlist cooperation by acknowledging the youth's expert knowledge about himself or herself. Explain the questions you will ask; for example, you can say, "I am going to ask you some questions about your past in order to learn more about you." The Typology Survey begins with basic identifying information about the adolescent and builds up (as does rapport) to more difficult questions. Be aware of the youth's comfort level throughout the assessment. Tell the adolescent to let you know of any uncomfortable feelings, since you can conduct this assessment in segments over several sessions. However, it is okay to periodically ask how the process feels, as not all youth will voluntarily disclose if feeling uncomfortable. Maintain an open conversation while administering this assessment; it will encourage the youth to speak more freely. You may ask questions, make some light comments to relax the adolescent, and take breaks. Once you begin the assessment, write down all responses in the spaces provided in the form. Be sure to complete all areas, even if they seem irrelevant. Remember that this information is essential for later completing your case conceptualization, as well as providing effective therapy. Next, we briefly review the 12 sections of the Typology Survey. The entire protocol is presented in appendix A.

Guidelines for Completing the Typology Survey

I. **Identifying Information:** Record the youth's identifying personal data: name, date of birth/age, ethnicity, date of admission to treatment.

II. **Family Information:** Record information regarding the youth's family of origin. Include whether the youth is living with an adoptive, foster, or biological family. It is important to identify any young children and/or any extended family living in the home.

III. **Substance Abuse History:** Record substance abuse history. If there is significant drug history (more than just trying a drug or alcohol once) make a referral to a chemical dependency department in your area for an in-depth assessment and a specific chemical dependency treatment.

IV. **Medical:** Record relevant medical history, including childhood head trauma, central nervous system damage, and/or mother's drug and alcohol use during pregnancy. These are all known to have adverse effects on a person's ability to function effectively.

V. **Educational:** Record relevant educational history, including special education services, academic goals, and any vocational or independent living training.

VI. **Emotional:** Record relevant history regarding suicidal, homicidal, or elopement ideation, gestures, or attempts. Include sleep, appetite, mood, bedwetting, and so forth, as well as any previous treatment, counseling, youth programs, or hospitalization.

VII. **Physiological:** First, describe one situation during which the youth became angry; then identify each physiological change that the youth experienced; last, rank them in the order in which they occurred.

VIII. **Interpersonal Relationships/Social History:** Record relevant interpersonal history and sexual history. Include what the youth likes to do for fun and what the youth typically does during free time. Sexual history is important in order to gain an understanding of the youth's sexual habits, preferences, and deviancy (if any). Many times adolescents do not recognize that what he or she considers to be normal, consensual experiences are actually offenses.

IX. **Behavioral Data:** Fill in the worksheet provided for this section. Include all behavior disorders or problem behaviors, such as fire setting, cruelty to animals, or other offenses. If there are sex offenses, include the victim's name, relationship, age of youth and victim at the time of the offense, number of times the offense occurred, description of the offense, how the youth persuaded the victim to go along with the offense, how the youth was caught, and any related criminal charges. Use a separate section for each victim. There are sections for seven victims. Copy this worksheet for additional victims. Please note the space provided for the youth's responses, interview(s) with parent/guardian, and chart review. It is important that you complete all columns for each victim.

X. **History of Physical and Sexual Abuse:** Fill in the worksheets, one for physical abuse and one for sexual abuse. Include the perpetrator's name (if available), relationship, age of the youth at the onset of the abuse, duration of the abuse, perpetrator's age, number of times the abuse occurred, description of the abuse, how the perpetrator persuaded the youth to go along with the abuse (if sexual), how the abuse was discovered, what was done about it, whether the abuse has been reported, and the outcome of reporting the abuse. If the abuse has not been reported, consult your clinical coordinator and/or state reporting regulations and report the abuse.

XI. **History of Other Abuse or Trauma:** Identify history of emotional abuse. Emotional abuse of a child is defined as poor treatment including invalidation; calling the child names; making statements that the child is worthless, is a bad person, deserves to be abused, or will never amount to anything; and making similar hurtful remarks. It is important to determine whether the abuse has been reported and what the outcome of the reporting was. Neglect is defined as failing to provide and/or care for a child. This can be in terms of food, shelter, clothing, attention, love, parenting, and similar needs. Include any other trauma, such as the death of someone close, having his/her life threatened, witnessing violence, family stressors, gang involvement, and any survival skills the youth needed and used to survive in the home environment.

XII. **Expectations of Treatment:** Include what the youth would like to do differently after completing treatment goals for the next year, willingness to be involved in family therapy (if appropriate), and what the youth would like to be different about himself or herself. It is also useful to get the youth's level of commitment to the process in order to establish a foundation for treatment.

Again, please refer to appendix A for a copy of the complete Typology Survey. Next, we discuss the Reactive-Proactive Scale.

The Reactive-Proactive Scale

After completing the Typology Survey, the next step in the MDT process is to explore the adolescent's fears in order to provide insight into underlying traumas. This is accomplished by the Fear Assessments, discussed in chapter 5. Through evaluation of the adolescent's reactive aggression, the Reactive-Proactive Scale helps you determine the appropriate Fear Assessment to use with the youth.

Reactive-Proactive Scale

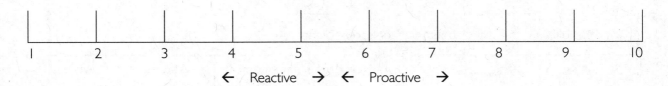

© 2009 Jack A. Apsche, EdD, ABPP

The 20 questions for the Reactive-Proactive Scale are presented on the next page, followed by the Reactive-Proactive Scale Scoring Chart and the Reactive-Proactive Scale Interpretation Key.

MDT Reactive-Proactive Scale

Name: _____ Date: _____

Answer the following questions about your adolescent client.

	Never	Sometimes	Almost Always	Always
1. Does the adolescent disclose past history including abuse, with minimal effort?	1	2	3	4
2. Does the adolescent express some difficulty with openness, and have difficulty verbalizing problems, such as above?	1	2	3	4
3. Does the adolescent avoid the term "fear" and have difficulty talking about feelings?	1	2	3	4
4. Can the adolescent identify any issues or problems with himself/herself?	1	2	3	4
5. Does the adolescent blame others for his/her problems?	1	2	3	4
6. Does the adolescent view life as "difficulties" rather than fears or problems?	1	2	3	4
7. Does the adolescent perceive emotional problems as something that others have?	1	2	3	4
8. Can the adolescent express his/her emotions about a past and current problem?	1	2	3	4
9. Does the adolescent often appear to take advantage of others verbally?	1	2	3	4
10. Does the adolescent engage in threats or intimidation of weaker people?	1	2	3	4
11. Does the adolescent fight based on repeated perceived threats from others?	1	2	3	4

	1	2	3	4
12. Has the adolescent been observed teasing or making fun of others out of the view of authority figures or care providers?	1	2	3	4
13. Does the adolescent "flash" his/her anger based on perceived slights or threats?	1	2	3	4
14. Does the adolescent take things from weaker adolescents because he/she can?	1	2	3	4
15. Does the adolescent have a history of physical abuse or "harsh discipline"?	1	2	3	4
16. Was the onset of behavioral problems for the adolescent by age six or prior?	1	2	3	4
17. Does the adolescent perceive that he/she was neglected by his/her parents or a caregiver as a child?	1	2	3	4
18. Will the adolescent get angry and attack others in front of a caregiver or authority figure?	1	2	3	4
19. Does the adolescent have difficulty relating to peers?	1	2	3	4
20. Does the adolescent always seem to be in the area of trouble, but never "gets caught?"	1	2	3	4

© 2009 Jack A. Apsche, EdD, ABPP

After completing the 20 questions, use the Reactive-Proactive Scale Scoring Chart below, showing which questions indicate proactive or reactive tendencies. To complete, write the score next to the number of each question provided, then figure the total for each column. Next, look at the Reactive-Proactive Scale Interpretation Key and use the total score to determine where to plot your client on the reactive to proactive continuum. The place you plot the score on the continuum suggests what specific Fear Assessment to use based on the youth's tendencies of reactive or proactive aggression. The scoring and interpretation charts are provided next.

Reactive-Proactive Scale Scoring Chart

Reactive	Proactive
1 _____	2 _____
4 _____	3 _____
8 _____	5 _____
11 _____	6 _____
13 _____	7 _____
15 _____	9 _____
16 _____	10 _____
17 _____	12 _____
18 _____	14 _____
19 _____	20 _____

TOTAL =

© 2009 Jack A. Apsche, EdD, ABPP

Reactive-Proactive Scale Interpretation Key

Total Score Reactive	Total Score Proactive
10–16 = 1	10–16 = 6
17–22 = 2	17–22 = 7
23–28 = 3	23–28 = 8
29–34 = 4	29–34 = 9
35–40 = 5	35–40 = 10

Select and plot the higher number score from the total of each column in the Reactive and Proactive Interpretation Key.

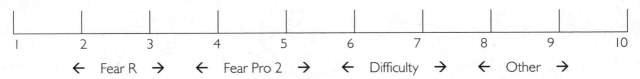

© 2009 Jack A. Apsche, EdD, ABPP

Results of the Reactive-Proactive Scale clearly guide you as to which Fear Assessment to administer to the adolescent.

Summary

In this chapter you were introduced to three MDT assessments: Beliefs about Therapeutic Alliance, the Typology Survey, and the Reactive-Proactive Scale. Through them, you begin your journey in the discovery of the function of the adolescent's behaviors, beliefs, fears, and emotions. We know that it's a lot to take in and, for some of you, it may even be a different therapeutic perspective. But please keep an open mind and take MDT a step at a time. An old Persian proverb tells us, "All things seem difficult until they are easy." As you read this book, you can go back and review the concepts and assessments at any time, until you are truly comfortable with them. The MDT Case Conceptualization process will help you better understand and more effectively treat the angry, aggressive, and oppositional adolescent. We are certain that this process will help you become a more effective and successful therapist. The next chapter explores the Fear Assessments—taking you closer to the crux of the adolescent's challenging behaviors. Now, as you prepare for chapter 5, breathe and be mindful of yourself and your progress as an MDT clinician.

Chapter 5

Discovering the Fear Assessments

The series of MDT assessments known as the Fear Assessments were specifically designed to identify underlying anxiety in the adolescent. This anxiety is manifested behaviorally through experiential avoidance (Hayes et al., 1999) and, if left untreated, can become a lifelong impediment to a positive, quality life. This underlying anxiety or internalizing disorder often fuels the fear response in reactive adolescents, which can lead to aggressive behavior. There are four Fear Assessments to choose from in MDT methodology for treatment of adolescents. Each Fear Assessment explores the client's responses to trauma and other threats experienced in his/her life as they affect the youth's well-being. That is, the assessments measure the relationship between the youth and his or her fear(s) and/or trauma. The fears endorsed by the adolescent activate experiential avoidance and, therefore, their identification is a critical component for completing the MDT case conceptualization. There are also four other types of Fear Assessments relevant to Family MDT which are beyond the scope of this book. The four individual Fear Assessments we introduce here are (1) Fear Assessment – Revised, (2) Fear Assessment – Revised II, (3) Difficulty Assessment – Revised, and (4) Difficulty Assessment for Others – Revised. Copies of all four individual Fear Assessments are included in this chapter.

Each 60-item Fear Assessment examines five subcategories of fear. These subcategories or indexes were designed to be sensitive to the detection of trauma, and each one represents part of a criterion for post-traumatic stress disorder (PTSD): Personal Reactive–External Index, Personal Reactive–Internal/Self-Concept Index, Environmental Index, Physical Index, and Abuse Index.

- The **Personal Reactive–External** index examines the adolescent's response to perceived external stimuli. This fear has a relationship with externalizing disorders as it evaluates the adolescent's responses to "perceived" external threats.

- The **Personal Reactive–Internal/Self-Concept** index examines the adolescent's internalization of trauma, or how the adolescent responds to the anxiety-related stimuli. This fear appears to have a relationship with some internalizing disorders.

- The **Environmental** index examines the adolescent's response to the actual physical environment. It also identifies specific fears that may result in avoidance of places in the adolescent's life.

- The **Physical** index examines the adolescent's response to physical stimuli that may account for the youth's fear and avoidance of specific physical contact and proximity to others in his/her life.

- The **Abuse** index examines the adolescent's response to specific stimuli from his/her experience of abuse. This is indicative of specific fears related to trauma, neglect, and perceived or real pain from trauma.

Selecting the Fear Assessment

It is important for the clinician to understand the specific purpose of each of the Fear Assessments in order to choose the appropriate one for administration. Additionally, Fear Assessment results are an integral component of the MDT methodology, leading to the case conceptualization and to treatment. You determine which Fear Assessment to use based on the information obtained from the Typology Survey and the Reactive-Proactive Scale, taking special notice of the adolescent's trauma history, as well as his/her willingness to disclose personal information. Consider the following guidelines when selecting the Fear Assessment to administer. If the youth:

- has an extensive trauma history and is open to discussing his/her history, use the *Fear Assessment – Revised*.

- has a trauma history and some proactive tendencies but is not as open to discussion, use the *Fear Assessment – Revised – 2*.

- has some trauma history but is not open to discussing personal fears and anxieties, use the *Difficulty Assessment – Revised*.

- is not open to discussing personal issues and attempts to "fake good," use the *Difficulty Assessment for Others – Revised*.

The four individual MDT Fear Assessments are presented in their entirety on the following pages. We encourage you to take your time and familiarize yourself with each one before you proceed to the next section, Guidelines for Completing the Fear Assessment.

MODE DEACTIVATION THERAPY (MDT) FEAR ASSESSMENT – REVISED

Name: _____ Date: _____

Circle the number below that corresponds to the fear that you experience. Briefly provide specific information where requested.

	Never	Sometimes	Almost Always	Always
1. Fear of trusting anyone.	1	2	3	4
2. Fear of trusting males - younger, older, race _____.	1	2	3	4
3. Fear of trusting females - younger, older, race _____.	1	2	3	4
4. Fear of trusting relative - specific relative _____.	1	2	3	4
5. Fear of being home alone.	1	2	3	4
6. Fear of closed rooms.	1	2	3	4
7. Fear of showers or bathrooms. Be specific.	1	2	3	4
8. Fear of failing. Be specific, failing at what?	1	2	3	4
9. Fear someone will do something sexual. Who? The sexual behaviors I am afraid of are _____.	1	2	3	4
10. Fear of hurting someone. Who?	1	2	3	4
11. Fear of someone hurting me.	1	2	3	4
12. Fear that I did something wrong.	1	2	3	4
13. Fear of not being smart.	1	2	3	4
14. Fear of nighttime.	1	2	3	4
15. Fear of being weak.	1	2	3	4
16. Fear of not being masculine/ feminine enough.	1	2	3	4
17. Fear of being gay/lesbian.	1	2	3	4

	1	2	3	4
18. Fear of dying. How? _____.	1	2	3	4
19. Fear of my anger.	1	2	3	4
20. Fear that someone will beat me up.	1	2	3	4
21. Fear of someone knowing the secret.	1	2	3	4
22. Fear that I caused the problem.	1	2	3	4
23. Fear that no one will believe me.	1	2	3	4
24. Fear that I have no one to talk to.	1	2	3	4
25. Fear of being used by others.	1	2	3	4
26. Fear of not being strong enough to get away.	1	2	3	4
27. Fear of being caught.	1	2	3	4
28. Fear that people will know by looking at me that I've done something wrong.	1	2	3	4
29. Fear that I will live.	1	2	3	4
30. Fear that I am sick and they will find out.	1	2	3	4
31. Fear of a specific place: _____.	1	2	3	4
32. Fear of being emotionally intimate.	1	2	3	4
33. Fear of crowds.	1	2	3	4
34. Fear of being alone.	1	2	3	4
35. Fear that I will die young.	1	2	3	4
36. Fear that I will be physically hurt for no reason.	1	2	3	4
37. Fear that something is wrong with me.	1	2	3	4
38. Fear of never being "normal."	1	2	3	4
39. Fear of my feelings.	1	2	3	4
40. Fear that I will never feel good.	1	2	3	4
41. Fear of talking with someone about my sexual abuse.	1	2	3	4

42. Fear of being in a crowded room.	1	2	3	4
43. Fear of being touched by someone that I don't know well.	1	2	3	4
44. Fear of being alone with adults that look like my abuser.	1	2	3	4
45. Fear of seeing the person who abused me.	1	2	3	4
46. Fear of reading about the person who abused me.	1	2	3	4
47. Fear of someone coming up behind me.	1	2	3	4
48. Fear of someone standing too close to me.	1	2	3	4
49. Fear of seeing someone the same size and race of my abuser.	1	2	3	4
50. Fear of being locked or restricted in a room.	1	2	3	4
51. Fear of wearing clothes similar to those worn when I was abused.	1	2	3	4
52. Fear of seeing and hearing about an assault on TV.	1	2	3	4
53. Fear of having sexual contact.	1	2	3	4
54. Fear of having physical contact.	1	2	3	4
55. Fear of losing control.	1	2	3	4
56. Fear of talking to strangers.	1	2	3	4
57. Fear of going to the place where I was abused.	1	2	3	4
58. Fear of confronting my abuser.	1	2	3	4
59. Fear of talking to a therapist about my abuse.	1	2	3	4
60. Fear that my abuser will get me again.	1	2	3	4

MODE DEACTIVATION THERAPY (MDT) FEAR ASSESSMENT – REVISED – 2

Name: _____ Date: _____

Circle the number below that corresponds to the fear that you experience. Briefly provide specific information where requested.

	Never	Sometimes	Almost Always	Always
1. Fear of trusting anyone.	1	2	3	4
2. Fear of trusting males - younger, older, race _____ .	1	2	3	4
3. Fear of trusting females - younger, older, race _____ .	1	2	3	4
4. Fear of trusting relatives - specific relative: _____ .	1	2	3	4
5. Fear of being betrayed by a trusted friend.	1	2	3	4
6. Fear of being alone in a room.	1	2	3	4
7. Fear of never getting out of the system.	1	2	3	4
8. Fear of failing. Be specific, failing at what?	1	2	3	4
9. Fear of someone thinking I am weak.	1	2	3	4
10. Fear of hurting someone.	1	2	3	4
11. Fear of someone hurting me emotionally.	1	2	3	4
12. Fear that I did something wrong.	1	2	3	4
13. Fear of not being as smart as others think I am.	1	2	3	4
14. Fear my family will give up on me.	1	2	3	4
15. Fear of being weaker inside than I want people to know.	1	2	3	4

16. Fear of not being masculine/ feminine enough.	1	2	3	4
17. Fear of having gay or lesbian thoughts sometimes.	1	2	3	4
18. Fear of never getting what I really want in life.	1	2	3	4
19. Fear of my anger.	1	2	3	4
20. Fear that someone will get me someday.	1	2	3	4
21. Fear of someone knowing my secret.	1	2	3	4
22. Fear that I caused the problem.	1	2	3	4
23. Fear my life is out of control.	1	2	3	4
24. Fear that I have no one to talk honestly with.	1	2	3	4
25. Fear of being used by others.	1	2	3	4
26. Fear of not being strong enough to deal with my hidden problems.	1	2	3	4
27. Fear of being caught.	1	2	3	4
28. Fear that people will know by looking at me, I've done something wrong.	1	2	3	4
29. Fear that I will never really be able to be close to anyone.	1	2	3	4
30. Fear that I am sick and they will find out.	1	2	3	4
31. Fear of not being really believed.	1	2	3	4
32. Fear of never trusting anyone fully.	1	2	3	4
33. Fear of crowds.	1	2	3	4
34. Fear of being alone in the world forever.	1	2	3	4
35. Fear that I will die young.	1	2	3	4
36. Fear that I will be physically hurt for no reason.	1	2	3	4

37. Fear that something is wrong with me.	1	2	3	4
38. Fear that I am becoming a criminal.	1	2	3	4
39. Fear of never feeling good again.	1	2	3	4
40. Fear that I will never be the person who I want to be.	1	2	3	4
41. Fear of my own thoughts.	1	2	3	4
42. Fear of being "set up by someone."	1	2	3	4
43. Fear of being accused of something that I did not do.	1	2	3	4
44. Fear of being trapped somewhere with no way out.	1	2	3	4
45. Fear of seeing someone get hurt for no reason.	1	2	3	4
46. Fear of going out in the world by myself without the support of my family.	1	2	3	4
47. Fear of someone coming up behind me.	1	2	3	4
48. Fear of someone standing too close to me.	1	2	3	4
49. Fear of seeing someone get hurt in front of me.	1	2	3	4
50. Fear of being locked or restricted in a room.	1	2	3	4
51. Fear of being shot or stabbed.	1	2	3	4
52. Fear of seeing and/or hearing murders in my neighborhood.	1	2	3	4
53. Fear of never being loved the way I want.	1	2	3	4
54. Fear of never being real about my deep problems.	1	2	3	4
55. Fear of totally losing control of myself.	1	2	3	4

56. Fear of being honest with myself.	1	2	3	4
57. Fear of being myself to people I don't really know well.	1	2	3	4
58. Fear of being verbally criticized in a condescending manner.	1	2	3	4
59. Fear of something I did not do will hurt me.	1	2	3	4
60. Fear that someone will get me if I let my guard down.	1	2	3	4

© 2009 Jack A. Apsche, EdD, ABPP

MODE DEACTIVATION THERAPY (MDT) DIFFICULTY ASSESSMENT – REVISED

Name: _____ Date: _____

Circle the number below that corresponds to the difficulty that you experience. Briefly provide specific information where requested.

	Never	**Sometimes**	**Almost Always**	**Always**
1. Difficulty trusting anyone.	1	2	3	4
2. Difficulty trusting males - younger, older, race _____ .	1	2	3	4
3. Difficulty trusting females - younger, older, race _____ .	1	2	3	4
4. Difficulty trusting relatives - specific relative: _____ .	1	2	3	4
5. Worried about being betrayed by a trusted friend.	1	2	3	4
6. Difficulty with being alone in a room.	1	2	3	4
7. Worried that I will never get out of the system.	1	2	3	4
8. Worried that I will fail. Be specific, fail at what?	1	2	3	4
9. Worried that someone will think I am weak.	1	2	3	4
10. Worried that I'll hurt someone.	1	2	3	4
11. Worried that someone will hurt me emotionally.	1	2	3	4
12. Worried that I did something wrong.	1	2	3	4
13. Difficulty with not being as smart as others think I am.	1	2	3	4
14. Worried that my family will give up on me.	1	2	3	4

15. Worried that I am weaker inside than I want people to know.	1	2	3	4
16. Worried by thoughts of not being masculine/feminine enough.	1	2	3	4
17. Difficulty with having sexual thoughts about males/females.	1	2	3	4
18. Worried that I'll never have what I really want in life.	1	2	3	4
19. My anger worries me.	1	2	3	4
20. Difficulty thinking that someone will get me someday.	1	2	3	4
21. Worried about someone knowing my secret.	1	2	3	4
22. Worried that I caused the problem.	1	2	3	4
23. Worried that my life is out of control.	1	2	3	4
24. Worried that I have no one to talk honestly with.	1	2	3	4
25. Difficulty with being used by others.	1	2	3	4
26. Worried about not being strong enough to deal with my hidden problems.	1	2	3	4
27. Worried about being caught.	1	2	3	4
28. Worried people will know by looking at me, I've done something wrong.	1	2	3	4
29. Worried that I will never really be able to be close to anyone.	1	2	3	4
30. Worried that I am sick and "they" will find out.	1	2	3	4
31. Difficulty with not being really believed.	1	2	3	4
32. Difficulty of never trusting anyone fully.	1	2	3	4
33. Being scared of crowds.	1	2	3	4

	1	2	3	4
34. Difficulty with being in the world forever.	1	2	3	4
35. Worried about thoughts of dying young.	1	2	3	4
36. Worried I will be physically hurt for no reason.	1	2	3	4
37. Worried that something is wrong with me.	1	2	3	4
38. Worried I am becoming a criminal.	1	2	3	4
39. Worried about never feeling good again.	1	2	3	4
40. Worried I will never be the person who I want to be.	1	2	3	4
41. Worried by my own thoughts.	1	2	3	4
42. Worried about being "set up by someone."	1	2	3	4
43. Worried about being accused of something that I did not do.	1	2	3	4
44. Difficulty with thinking about being trapped somewhere with no way out.	1	2	3	4
45. Worried about seeing someone hurt for no reason.	1	2	3	4
46. Scared of going out in the world by myself without the support of my family.	1	2	3	4
47. Someone coming up behind me makes me uncomfortable.	1	2	3	4
48. Difficulty with someone standing too close to me.	1	2	3	4
49. Worried about seeing someone hurt in front of me.	1	2	3	4
50. Difficulty with being locked or restricted in a room.	1	2	3	4
51. Worried that I'll be shot or stabbed.	1	2	3	4

52. Worried about seeing or hearing murders in my neighborhood.	1	2	3	4
53. Difficulty with never being loved the way I want.	1	2	3	4
54. Difficulty with never being real about my deep problems.	1	2	3	4
55. Difficulty with totally losing control of myself.	1	2	3	4
56. Difficulty with being honest with myself.	1	2	3	4
57. Difficulty with being myself to people I don't really know well.	1	2	3	4
58. Difficulty with being verbally criticized in a condescending manner.	1	2	3	4
59. Worried that something I did not do will hurt me.	1	2	3	4
60. Worried that someone will get me if I let my guard down.	1	2	3	4

MODE DEACTIVATION THERAPY (MDT) DIFFICULTY ASSESSMENT FOR OTHERS – REVISED

Name: _____ Date: _____

Circle the number below that corresponds to the difficulty that you perceive others experience. Briefly provide specific information where requested.

	Never	Sometimes	Almost Always	Always
1. Others in my position might have difficulty trusting anyone.	1	2	3	4
2. Many people might have difficulty trusting males - younger, older, race _____ .	1	2	3	4
3. Many people might have difficulty trusting females - younger, older, race _____ .	1	2	3	4
4. A lot of my peers might have difficulty trusting relatives - specific relative: _____ .	1	2	3	4
5. Other people with my background may be worried of being betrayed by a trusted friend.	1	2	3	4
6. Some people like me could have difficulty being alone in a room.	1	2	3	4
7. Most people would be worried that they will never get out of the system.	1	2	3	4
8. Most people would be worried that they will fail. Be specific, what would they fail at?	1	2	3	4
9. Many people are worried that someone will think that they are weak.	1	2	3	4
10. Some people would be worried that they will hurt someone.	1	2	3	4
11. Others would be worried that someone will hurt them emotionally.	1	2	3	4

	1	2	3	4
12. Others may be worried that they did something wrong.	1	2	3	4
13. Some people have difficulty with not being as smart as others think they are.	1	2	3	4
14. Many adolescents in my position would be worried that their family would give up on them.	1	2	3	4
15. Many of my peers are worried that they are weaker inside than they want people to know.	1	2	3	4
16. Thoughts of not being masculine/ feminine enough worry some people.	1	2	3	4
17. Some people are worried about having sexual thoughts of males/females.	1	2	3	4
18. Some of my peers are worried that they'll never have what they really want in life.	1	2	3	4
19. Others are worried by their anger.	1	2	3	4
20. Some adolescents have difficulty thinking that someone will get them someday.	1	2	3	4
21. Many people are worried about someone knowing their secret.	1	2	3	4
22. Some of my peers are worried that they caused the problem.	1	2	3	4
23. Other people are worried that their life is out of control.	1	2	3	4
24. Some people may be worried that they have no one to talk honestly with.	1	2	3	4
25. Many people have difficulty with being used by others.	1	2	3	4
26. Some people are worried about not being strong enough to deal with their hidden problems.	1	2	3	4

27. The thought of being caught worries some people.	1	2	3	4
28. Many of my peers worry that people will know by looking at them that they have done something wrong.	1	2	3	4
29. Others in my position might be worried that they will never be able to be close to anyone.	1	2	3	4
30. Other people would be worried that they are sick and someone will find out.	1	2	3	4
31. Others in my position might have difficulty with not being believed.	1	2	3	4
32. Other people with my background have difficulty never trusting anyone fully.	1	2	3	4
33. Some people are scared of crowds.	1	2	3	4
34. People in my position have difficulty with being alone in the world forever.	1	2	3	4
35. Thoughts of dying young worry many people in my position.	1	2	3	4
36. Some of my peers are worried they will be physically hurt for no reason.	1	2	3	4
37. Other people are worried that something is wrong with them.	1	2	3	4
38. Other adolescents in my position may be worried that they are becoming criminals.	1	2	3	4
39. Many of my peers are worried that they will never feel good again.	1	2	3	4
40. Some people are worried that they will never be the person they want to be.	1	2	3	4
41. Some of my peers have thoughts that worry them.	1	2	3	4

42. I know people who are worried of being "set up by someone."	1	2	3	4
43. Others in my position may be worried of being accused of something that they did not do.	1	2	3	4
44. Other people with my background have difficulties with thinking about being trapped somewhere with no way out.	1	2	3	4
45. Some people are worried about seeing someone hurt for no reason.	1	2	3	4
46. Other people with my background may be scared of going out in the world without the support of their family.	1	2	3	4
47. Some people are uncomfortable when someone comes up behind them.	1	2	3	4
48. Many of my peers have difficulty with someone standing too close to them.	1	2	3	4
49. Many adolescents are worried about seeing someone hurt in front of them.	1	2	3	4
50. Some people like me have difficulties of being locked or restricted in a room.	1	2	3	4
51. Many people with my background would be worried that they'll be shot or stabbed.	1	2	3	4
52. Seeing or hearing murders in the neighborhood would worry some people.	1	2	3	4
53. People with a similar background have difficulties with never being loved the way they want.	1	2	3	4

54. Others in my position might have difficulty with never being real about their deep problems.	1	2	3	4
55. Many adolescents in my position have difficulty with totally losing control of themselves.	1	2	3	4
56. Other people have difficulty with being honest with themselves.	1	2	3	4
57. Many people with my background have difficulty with being themselves to people they don't really know well.	1	2	3	4
58. Some of my peers have difficulty with being verbally criticized in a condescending manner.	1	2	3	4
59. Others have difficulty with thinking that something they did not do will hurt them.	1	2	3	4
60. Others with my background would have difficulty that someone will get them if they let their guard down.	1	2	3	4

© 2009 Jack A. Apsche, EdD, ABPP

Guidelines for Completing the Fear Assessments

All Fear Assessments are completed according to the same process: first requiring a clinician's evaluation, followed by a clinician and adolescent collaboration. That is, after you determine the appropriate type of Fear Assessment to use, but before administering it to the adolescent, review the instrument and endorse the fears that are valid for the youth according to behaviors observed, verbalized, and documented. In other words, identify fears you believe to be true for the youth based on his or her behavior, not fears you believe the youth will endorse.

The next step in the administration of a Fear Assessment is to meet with the adolescent during one or more sessions (as needed) to jointly fill out the instrument. It becomes the springboard for a conversation with the youth about his/her fears, with you writing down the adolescent's responses on the Fear Assessment form. Highlight or circle in a different color ink to differentiate the youth's responses from yours.

As previously indicated, all Fear Assessments follow the same guidelines. First, explain the response scale to the adolescent. This begins to engage the adolescent and make him or her more comfortable with the process in general. The adolescent can endorse the fears with "Sometimes," "Almost Always," or "Always," or may not endorse them at all by responding "Never." For example, explain the questions you will ask by saying, "I am going to ask you some questions about how you feel about certain situations." And explain the scale of responses by saying, "Tell me if you fear this 'Sometimes,' 'Almost always,' 'Always,' or 'Never.'"

It is important to be aware that the adolescent may process on a concrete level and fail to endorse a fear if it is not actually being experienced at that time. Therefore, it is critical to explain that fears can be present on different occasions; in addition, it is helpful to explore scenarios together to identify the presence of a fear during other situations. Some adolescents feel that they are "better" since participating in treatment and, as a result, will under-endorse fears. We recommend that you ask the youth to also identify fears experienced prior to treatment. Therefore, it may be beneficial to phrase the fears in the past tense to further clarify the concept of previous fears.

Be sure to explore the fears you highlighted with the adolescent, discussing your reasons if necessary. This is important! If he/she does not endorse a fear that you have highlighted, spend time clarifying what the fear means and how his or her behavior suggests endorsement. However, although you need to explain the context and/or meaning of the fear, do not coerce the adolescent into endorsing a fear; simply explore the fear together.

Use words that are comfortable for the adolescent. If he/she reacts to the word "fear," use words like "anxious," "nervous," "uncomfortable," "hard time," "difficulty," "dread," "panic," "fright," or "horror." For example, ask whether the adolescent "worries" or has "difficulty" with bedtime or whether "_____ ever bothers" him/her. Sometimes an adolescent will require prompting to accurately endorse responses. Ascertain the youth's definition of words like "trust" or "retaliation." Use real-life examples and/or scenarios to clarify questions and concepts. Rephrase questions so they resonate with the adolescent. For example, "You are standing on the corner near your house or in the hall at school, and all of a sudden someone is behind you, do you feel anxious, worried, nervous…?" Or "It's getting dark, it's hygiene time, and staff directs you to go to the shower. What is your fear, worry, or anxiety level?" In other words, use your clinician skills to build rapport and trust with the adolescent as you navigate together through the MDT process.

Some adolescents may find the response scale too restricting, so it could be useful to begin each assessment question by asking whether the fear is present or not. If he/she endorses the fear, you can then identify the frequency or intensity of the fear. Keep in mind that disclosing fears exposes vulnerability and it is natural to protect that vulnerability by reporting fears as occurring "Sometimes" or even "Never." This is often the case with resistant and/or severely abused adolescents, as they attempt to protect themselves by hiding their fears from others. If you notice predominantly "Never" or "Sometimes" responses, review the fears you highlighted prior to administering the assessment to the adolescent. Look at the pattern of responses. Again, it is important for you to explore fears that you believe to be true, based on the presence or history of behaviors. Share your reasons for believing the fear to be true with the adolescent and discuss the discrepancy in your responses.

Although most adolescents will respond to the Fear Assessments directly, there may be some who don't respond at all. If an adolescent doesn't respond, first, simply attempt to talk about the general reasons for the Fear Assessment and then end the session. Another strategy we suggest is to engage the adolescent in a mindfulness exercise (chapter 11) and afterward perhaps take a break. If the youth continues to refuse when you suggest that he/she resume the session with a mindfulness activity, end the session. You might want to attempt to administer the Fear Assessment at a later date. In that case, begin the next session with a brief mindfulness exercise and try administering the Fear Assessment again. With very reluctant or hostile adolescents, you can also use the Difficulty Assessment for Others – Revised. This assessment can be described to the adolescent as one that will give you information on other adolescents with a history of similar experiences. If the adolescent continues to refuse to participate, you can still elicit some responses from the youth based on his/her history and then prompt him/her to successful completion, or approximation of completion, of the Fear Assessment. Ask the adolescent for help: You can say, "I really need your help because you are the expert on your life." It is important that you communicate that your only motive is to make this process right and without the adolescent's help you are helpless to make anything right. We have found that when you honestly and sincerely enlist the adolescent's aid and earnestly empower him/her as an individual, the client collaborates with the clinician. Remember that angry, aggressive, and oppositional adolescents have a history of one-down relationships with adults, including their parents, teachers, judges, and others with power over them. However, once empowered by the clinician through trust and respect, you begin the real process of collaboration with the youth.

Scoring and Interpretation of the Fear Assessments

The same scoring key is used for all Fear Assessments presented in this chapter. They were designed and based on the Fear Assessment – Revised, which was statistically validated for adolescents ages 14 to 17. During the scoring and interpretation of the Fear Assessments, three areas are reviewed: Life-Interfering Fears, Fear Assessment Subcategories, and Fear Assessment Total Score.

Life-Interfering Fears

Life-interfering fears are a critical area of concern and the crux of all Fear Assessments. They activate the adolescent's experiential avoidance, as well as his or her life-interfering beliefs, which can result in a variety of aberrant behaviors, such as anger, aggression, parasuicide, and isolation from others. This fear → avoids paradigm is discussed in chapter 8. It is important for the clinician to be cognizant of how particular life-interfering fears activate the adolescent's mode by presenting a perceived threat to his/her ability to function. These fears are the essential fears that drive some of the adolescent's behaviors and are to be addressed first when completing the MDT Case Conceptualization.

In the Fear Assessments, 21 life-interfering fears are identified, found in the following items: 1, 2, 3, 4, 8, 12, 15, 19, 21, 22, 23, 24, 25, 28, 30, 32, 34, 37, 39, 54, and 55. Each life-interfering fear is identified in the Fear Assessment – Life-Interfering Fears Worksheet presented next. To score the life-interfering fears, first look at the responses on the completed Fear Assessment for the items listed on the worksheet. Circle only "Almost Always" (3) or "Always" (4) responses on the worksheet as applicable.

After completing the Life-Interfering Fears Worksheet, review the results to identify patterns of fears influential in the adolescent's life and to increase your understanding of the adolescent. For example, items 1 through 4 identify the presence of trust issues and can provide insight about the adolescent's perception of trusting others. Or, for instance, if an adolescent endorses item 8 (fear of failing) with a 3 or a 4, it is clear that this individual may likely avoid situations where he/she could fail. This, in essence, indicates that the adolescent may live his/her life trying to avoid the painful feelings that are associated with failing, and may not be able to live life in any productive or meaningful manner. Hence, a life-interfering fear activates life-interfering beliefs, causing behaviors that negatively impact the adolescent's potential for living a safe, high-quality life. Anger, aggression, self-injuring actions, and substance abuse are all behaviors correlated to the avoidance of feelings associated with failure. Use the following worksheet to identify which of the 21 life-interfering fears your adolescent presents.

MDT FEAR ASSESSMENT – LIFE-INTERFERING FEARS WORKSHEET

Name: _____ Date: _____

Fear Assessment Type: _____

Circle the 3 or 4 level responses obtained in the Fear Assessment to the items below. Put a check mark in the box next to the fears identified.

Fear Assessment Items	Fear	Almost Always	Always	Fears
1	Trusting anyone	3	4	☐
2	Trusting males	3	4	☐
3	Trusting females	3	4	☐
4	Trusting relatives	3	4	☐
8	Failing	3	4	☐
12	Did something wrong	3	4	☐
15	Being weak	3	4	☐
19	My anger	3	4	☐
21	Someone knowing my secret	3	4	☐
22	Causing the problem	3	4	☐
23	No one will believe me or my life is out of control	3	4	☐
24	Have no one to talk to	3	4	☐
25	Fear of being used by others	3	4	☐
28	People will know by looking at me that I've done something wrong	3	4	☐
30	I am sick and they will find out	3	4	☐
32	Being emotionally intimate	3	4	☐
34	Being alone	3	4	☐
37	Something is wrong with me	3	4	☐
39	My feelings	3	4	☐

| 54 | Having physical contact or being honest with others | 3 | 4 | ☐ |
| 55 | Fear of losing control of self | 3 | 4 | ☐ |

© 2009 Jack A. Apsche, EdD, ABPP

Fear Assessment Subcategories

As previously indicated, the Fear Assessments explore five subcategories of fears and trauma, or perceived trauma, in the adolescent. These are labeled the Personal Reactive–External Index, Personal Reactive–Internal/Self-Concept Index, Environmental Index, Physical Index, and Abuse Index. Fear Assessment results yield (1) individual mean scores for each subcategory, and (2) a total Fear Assessment score. These scores identify areas to address in treatment, as well as provide an indication of the level of trauma present in the adolescent. The specific items relevant to each subcategory are listed below; bold numbers at the end indicate the number of items in each subcategory.

(1) Personal Reactive–External Index (PRE)

1, 2, 3, 4, 8, 12, 19, 21, 22, 23, 24, 27, 28, 30, 54, 55 **(16)**

(2) Personal Reactive–Internal/Self-Concept Index (PRI/SC)

13, 15, 16, 17, 25, 29, 32, 34, 35, 36, 37, 38, 39, 40, 49, 56 **(16)**

(3) Environmental Index (E)

5, 6, 7, 31, 33, 42, 50 **(7)**

(4) Physical Index (P)

9, 10, 11, 14, 18, 20, 26, 43, 47, 48, 53 **(11)**

(5) Abuse Index (A)

41, 44, 45, 46, 51, 52, 57, 58, 59, 60 **(10)**

To obtain the mean for each subcategory, use the worksheet provided below. First, fill in the score obtained in the assessment next to the items listed. Then, subtotal (add) the scores and then divide by the number of items in the category. For example, for the Abuse Index, add the responses then divide by 10. This will give you the individual mean score for the Abuse subcategory. To calculate the Fear Assessment Total Score, add all the individual subcategory means (PRE + PRI/SC + E + P + A) obtained through the procedure described in the above paragraph.

The interpretation of subcategory means and total Fear Assessment scores is as follows:

1. If the mean score is above 2.0, this is a significant area of fear that will need to be addressed in therapy.

2. If the mean score is above 3.0 total or in subcategories, it is an indication of trauma. Often a 3.0 or above is predictive of possible PTSD or acute stress disorder.

MDT FEAR ASSESSMENT SUBCATEGORY SCORING GRID

Name: _____ Date: _____

Fear Assessment Type: _____

1. PERSONAL–REACTIVE EXTERNAL INDEX (PRE)

Item	Score	Item	Score	Item	Score	
1		19		28		
2		21		30		
3		22		54		
4		23		55		
8		24				
12		27				
Subtotals		+		+		÷16 = PRE Mean

PERSONAL–REACTIVE INTERNAL/SELF-CONCEPT INDEX (PRI/SC)

Item	Score	Item	Score	Item	Score	
13		32		38		
15		34		39		
16		35		40		
17		36		49		
25		37		56		
29						
Subtotals		+		+		÷ 16 = PRI/SC Mean

ENVIRONMENTAL INDEX (E)

Item	Score	Item	Score	Item	Score	
5		31		50		
6		33				
7		42				
Subtotals		+		+		÷ 7 = E Mean

PHYSICAL INDEX (P)						
Item	Score	Item	Score	Item	Score	
9		18		47		
10		20		48		
11		26		53		
14		43				
Subtotals	+	+	=			÷ 11 = P Mean
ABUSE INDEX (A)						
Item	Score	Item	Score	Item	Score	
41		51		59		
44		52		60		
45		57				
46		58				
Subtotals		+		+		÷ 10 = A Mean
PRE + PRI/SC + E + P + A = Total Fear Assessment Score = _____						

Overall, the MDT Fear Assessments are empirically based instruments that help identify elements of internalizing disorders, such as anxiety, that may present as severe aberrant and dangerous behaviors in adolescents.

Summary

The Fear Assessment is a critical component of the MDT process. It identifies the fears that fuel many internalizing disorders and manifest themselves in externalizing disorders, such as anger, aggression, parasuicide, and substance abuse. You can learn a great deal about the adolescent from the Fear Assessments. To facilitate the smooth administration of Fear Assessments: relax; be patient and supportive of the adolescent; make eye contact when appropriate; be observant of reactions; clarify with real-life scenarios; take as many sessions as needed to complete the assessment; let the client provide his or her responses, and explore them together. Remember, collaboration is the key to success, so feel free to help the youth relax by introducing a mindfulness exercise. The next chapter presents the Compound Core Belief Questionnaire.

Chapter 6

The Compound Core Belief Questionnaire – S

The next MDT assessment is the Compound Core Belief Questionnaire – S (CCBQ-S), a 96-item instrument designed to provide an understanding of the adolescent's underlying beliefs and thoughts, as well as his or her subsequent perceptions and reactions to feelings. This chapter will guide you step-by-step through the administration, scoring, and interpretation of the CCBQ-S.[1] The instrument and worksheets are provided for your use.

Through the exploration of underlying beliefs, the clinician can identify those beliefs that can interfere with the adolescent's success in life and/or treatment. We have found that the client's underlying beliefs can lead to the development of particular life-threatening and treatment-interfering beliefs. These beliefs are identified through the Compound Core Belief Questionnaire so the clinician can address them in MDT treatment. But before guiding you through the different steps of the CCBQ-S, let us first clarify what we mean by (1) underlying, (2) life-threatening, and (3) treatment-interfering beliefs. *Underlying beliefs* are a series of beliefs and schemas that are formed throughout the adolescent's life, based on experiences and cognitions, that are influential in his/her perceptions and reactions to life events. *Life-threatening beliefs* are those beliefs that, as we have found through our research, have a relationship to high-risk behaviors. These high-risk behaviors include, but are not limited to, suicidal and parasuicidal behavior, substance abuse, and reckless aggression. *Treatment-interfering beliefs* are those beliefs that support avoidant behaviors that interfere with the adolescent's success in treatment; for example, lack of trust, suspicion and mistrust of adults and authority figures, confabulation, and isolation.

The CCBQ-S offers the clinician an opportunity to gather valuable information concerning beliefs endorsed by the adolescent in order to begin to assess and identify the presence of personality traits and how they need to be addressed in MDT treatment. The beliefs endorsed on the CCBQ-S are also used later in the MDT process to complete the Triggers, Fears, and Avoids (TFAB)

---

1   The CCBQ-S is the short version of the CCBQ. The standard form is available at http://www.theapscheinstitute.com under Assessment Sessions.

Compound Core Beliefs Correlation component of the Case Conceptualization (presented in chapter 8). The CCBQ-S identifies the presence of the following eight types of beliefs in the adolescent: antisocial personality beliefs, avoidant personality beliefs, borderline personality beliefs, conduct beliefs, dependent personality beliefs, histrionic personality beliefs, narcissistic personality beliefs, and obsessive-compulsive beliefs. These eight types of beliefs correlate with specific personality traits and behaviors characteristic of angry, aggressive, and oppositional adolescents. They usually present as clusters of more than one belief and provide a profile of the adolescent, as well as a blueprint for MDT treatment. A brief explanation of each belief is provided below:

I. **Antisocial personality beliefs** are related or congruent with an antisocial lifestyle.

II. **Avoidant personality beliefs** are related to the avoidance of participating in life in general and in particular, avoidance of school, social, and recreational activities.

III. **Borderline personality beliefs** are related to concurrent dichotomous beliefs—those that convey an inability to establish a sense of self and/or reflect a dysregulation in mood and interpersonal relationships.

IV. **Conduct beliefs** are related to problem and delinquent behaviors.

V. **Dependent personality beliefs** are related to a pattern of dependence in the adolescent.

VI. **Histrionic personality beliefs** are related to overly dramatic behavior and a need for constant support and attention.

VII. **Narcissistic personality beliefs** are related to self-centeredness and egocentrism.

VIII. **Obsessive-compulsive beliefs** are related to the need to control or engage in life rigidly or in a restricted manner, or to the need for repetitive behaviors.

Guidelines for Completing the CCBQ-S

The CCBQ-S is completed in a similar manner to the Fear Assessments, and in fact we recommend that you review the section in chapter 5 titled Guidelines for Completing the Fear Assessment, to refresh your memory about strategies for administering and creating rapport with the youth when using MDT assessments. Before presenting the CCBQ-S to the adolescent, go over the instrument and highlight beliefs that would reflect the adolescent's behavior and the background information recorded in the Typology Survey or obtained from other sources, such as parents or caregivers, as well as from the adolescent's chart. Remember to highlight responses that the adolescent's behaviors support—not those you believe he/she may endorse. Next, explore your highlighted beliefs with the youth and provide your rationale for your selections as necessary. Clarify with the client any discrepancies where you (the clinician) identified beliefs not acknowledged by the youth. This process sets in motion a dialogue between you and the adolescent and helps continue to build the rapport between clinician and client.

The CCBQ-S uses four levels of responses: "Sometimes," "Almost Always," "Always," and "Never." It is important to explore with the adolescent beliefs experienced in the past as well as those experienced in the present. You can do this by saying to the youth, "I want you to tell me about some of the beliefs you had before treatment." As the adolescent identifies a past belief, ask whether or not he/she experiences the belief in the present. If yes, guide the youth to determine the belief's intensity and frequency ("Sometimes," "Almost always," "Always," or "Never"). Remember to also ask about new beliefs that the adolescent may be experiencing in the present.

Completing the CCBQ-S is a collaborative, thoughtful process that not only provides the clinician with significant data about the youth but also begins to develop insight (or at minimum, awareness) in the adolescent as to how beliefs influence decisions and perceptions in his or her life. It may take several sessions to complete and/or discuss the CCBQ-S in order to establish the necessary foundation for MDT treatment. That's all right; take your time—remember that as you gather information, you are also building a therapeutic alliance with your client.

As you progress through the CCBQ-S, try to determine whether there's a pattern to the responses. As with the Fear Assessment, resistant and/or severely abused adolescents tend to provide predominantly "Never" or "Sometimes" responses. These adolescents attempt to protect themselves by not endorsing beliefs that they perceive may make them appear vulnerable to others.

The CCBQ-S is presented next to provide you with the opportunity to familiarize yourself with it before we guide you through the scoring and interpretation process. Each assessment item correlates to one of the eight types of beliefs explained at the beginning of the chapter. The particular belief is identified by the Roman numeral at the end of each item.

COMPOUND CORE BELIEFS QUESTIONNAIRE – S (CCBQ-S)

Name: _____   Date: _____

Please read the statements below and *circle how often you believe each one.*

			Never	Sometimes	Almost Always	Always
☐	TI	1. Everyone betrays my trust. I cannot trust anyone. (III)	1	2	3	4
		2. If I am not loved, I am unhappy. (IV)	1	2	3	4
		3. I am so exciting; others always want to be with me. (V)	1	2	3	4
☐	TI	4. I cannot trust others; they will hurt me. (VII)	1	2	3	4
		5. If I trust someone today, they will betray me later. (III)	1	2	3	4
		6. I am only fulfilled by being with a strong person. (IV)	1	2	3	4
		7. Others are critical; therefore they will reject me. (II)	1	2	3	4
		8. There is no problem if others don't know I did something. (I)	1	2	3	4
		9. Other people have hidden motives and want something from me. (VII)	1	2	3	4
		10. Whenever I hope, I will become disappointed. (III)	1	2	3	4
		11. Others make better decisions than I do; I cannot make up my mind. (IV)	1	2	3	4
☐	LT	12. When I feel something, it may be unpleasant. (II)	1	2	3	4
☐	TI	13. Unless you have a videotape of me, you cannot prove I did it. (I)	1	2	3	4
		14. If you criticize me, you are against me. (VI)	1	2	3	4

			1	2	3	4
		15. If I don't make myself known, others will not know how special I am. (V)	1	2	3	4
		16. Things never work out for me; I never get a break. (VIII)	1	2	3	4
☐	TI	17. If I am not on guard, others will take advantage of me. (VII)	1	2	3	4
		18. I am so brilliant and special, only a "gifted" few understand me. (VI)	1	2	3	4
		19. When I am bored, I need to become the center of attention. (V)	1	2	3	4
		20. If I give others the chance, they will hurt me. (VII)	1	2	3	4
☐	LT	21. When I am angry, my emotions are extreme and out of control. (III)	1	2	3	4
		22. Others are stronger and I need them to cope.	1	2	3	4
☐	TI	23. I am inadequate; I will do whatever I must to hide it. (II)	1	2	3	4
☐	TI	24. My "inner feelings" and intuition are all I need; rational thinking doesn't help. (V)	1	2	3	4
		25. When I get angry, my emotions go from annoyed to furious. (III)	1	2	3	4
		26. If I am afraid something will be unpleasant, I will avoid it. (II)	1	2	3	4
		27. Others are unreliable, will let me down, or reject me. I need to protect myself. (III)	1	2	3	4
		28. When others are paying attention to me, I am never bored. (V)	1	2	3	4
		29. Others may make demands, but I do things my way. (VIII)	1	2	3	4
☐	TI	30. If I let others know me, they will take advantage and hurt me. (VII)	1	2	3	4
☐	LT	31. When I hurt emotionally, I do whatever it takes to feel better. (III)	1	2	3	4

☐	LT	32. Anything is better than feeling unpleasant. (II)	1	2	3	4
		33. If I act silly and entertain people, they won't notice my weaknesses. (V)	1	2	3	4
		34. If I let others know information about me, they will use it against me. (VII)	1	2	3	4
		35. If others notice me, they will see my inadequacies. (II)	1	2	3	4
		36. People tell me or say things to me, and mean something else. (VII)	1	2	3	4
		37. Life at times feels like an endless series of disappointments followed by pain. (III)	1	2	3	4
☐	LT	38. If I feel bad, I can't control it. (II)	1	2	3	4
☐	TI	39. I can do what I want; consequences don't affect me directly unless I am caught. (I)	1	2	3	4
		40. Consequences only matter when I am caught. They are for others. (I)	1	2	3	4
☐	TI	41. If others think they can get away with taking advantage of me, they will use me and information about me. (VII)	1	2	3	4
		42. If I don't take what I want, I won't get what I need; and I deserve it. (I)	1	2	3	4
☐	LT	43. I try to control and not to show my grieving, loss, sadness, but eventually it comes out in a rush of emotions. (III)	1	2	3	4
		44. If I don't think about or deal with a problem, it is not real. (II)	1	2	3	4
		45. People are not worth being around if they criticize me. (II)	1	2	3	4
		46. My feelings about myself are so poor that I will do whatever I need to do to compensate for it. (III)	1	2	3	4
		47. Whenever I try to feel better, I make things worse and feel more pain eventually. (III)	1	2	3	4

			1	2	3	4
		48. If they ask me to do something I don't want to do, I'll pay them back. (VIII)	1	2	3	4
		49. I do it because I can; I deserve to get what I want. (I)	1	2	3	4
		50. Whenever I need someone, they are not there for me; there is no one I can count on. (III)	1	2	3	4
		51. Rules are for others. (VI)	1	2	3	4
		52. If people don't respond positively to me, they are not important. (V)	1	2	3	4
		53. I need to avoid situations in which I am the center of attention; I should be behind the scenes. (II)	1	2	3	4
		54. I don't have to follow the rules for other people. (VI)	1	2	3	4
		55. It is OK to do what I do as long as I get away with it. (I)	1	2	3	4
☐	TI	56. I would rather not try something new than fail at it. (II)	1	2	3	4
		57. I have every reason to expect wonderful things for myself, since I am so special. (VI)	1	2	3	4
☐	TI	58. I've been treated badly, so whatever I need to do to get what I need is OK. (I)	1	2	3	4
		59. My "gut" feelings tell what I need to do; that's more important than thinking through problems. (V)	1	2	3	4
		60. I never make decisions on my own; I always need support. (IV)	1	2	3	4
☐	LT	61. Unpleasant feelings usually escalate and then get out of control and get worse. (II)	1	2	3	4
		62. My needs are more important; others' needs shouldn't interfere. (VI)	1	2	3	4
		63. I will con people to get whatever I need; it's not a problem. (I)	1	2	3	4
		64. Since I am so talented and gifted, others should help me get what I want. (VI)	1	2	3	4

			1	2	3	4
		65. Others should not criticize me; if they do it's because they usually can't understand me. (VI)	1	2	3	4
☐	TI	66. If people don't care for themselves, whatever happens to them is their problem. (I)	1	2	3	4
		67. Circumstances dictate how I feel and behave. (V)	1	2	3	4
		68. When I am abandoned, I feel like life is over. (IV)	1	2	3	4
		69. If people do not show me respect and give me what I am entitled to, it is intolerable for me. (VI)	1	2	3	4
		70. Most of my relationships with people are extremely intimate, because people love to be around me or with me. (V)	1	2	3	4
		71. I am happiest when people pay attention to me. (V)	1	2	3	4
		72. I cannot handle my life without support. (IV)	1	2	3	4
☐	LT	73. I am needy and weak inside, no matter what others see. (IV)	1	2	3	4
☐	TI	74. I tell a girl/boy anything I need to get sex, or what I want. (I)	1	2	3	4
		75. I must be subservient to all in authority; I cannot make it on my own. (IV)	1	2	3	4
		76. I don't need to work to achieve; things should come my way because I deserve it. (VI)	1	2	3	4
		77. Whenever I end a relationship, I immediately find a new one. (IV)	1	2	3	4
		78. Most people are not as gifted as I am, and my behavior lets them know it. (VI)	1	2	3	4
		79. Whenever I am not getting attention, I am bored. (V)	1	2	3	4
☐	LT	80. Being alone is terrible. (IV)	1	2	3	4
		81. If I don't "take care" of them first, then they will get me. (I)	1	2	3	4

			1	2	3	4
		82. I cannot cope like others, I need support. (IV)	1	2	3	4
		83. Others' feelings are not as important as achieving a goal for myself. (VI)	1	2	3	4
☐	TI	84. If other people get any information on me, they will use it against me. (VII)	1	2	3	4
☐	TI	85. Other people expect too much from me. (VIII)	1	2	3	4
		86. If others are too bossy and demanding, I don't have to follow them. (VIII)	1	2	3	4
☐	TI	87. Authority figures tend to be controlling/demanding and act like they are in control. (VIII)	1	2	3	4
		88. Others always have hidden motives and I cannot really trust anyone. (VII)	1	2	3	4
		89. If I don't want to do something, my mood changes and I withdraw emotionally. (VIII)	1	2	3	4
		90. If I let others know "who I am," they'll know my weaknesses and use them against me. (VII)	1	2	3	4
☐	TI	91. I never like to show my anger directly but others know when I am angry. (VIII)	1	2	3	4
		92. Others should not tell me what to do; I will eventually do what I want anyway. (VIII)	1	2	3	4
		93. I have to keep myself from being dominated by authority figures, while gaining their acceptance and approval. (VIII)	1	2	3	4
		94. Others often attempt to get something over on me by exploiting or harming me in some way. (VII)	1	2	3	4
		95. I really am self-sufficient but I often need others' help to reach my goals. (VIII)	1	2	3	4
		96. Authority figures usually stifle my creativity and prevent my progress toward goals. (VIII)	1	2	3	4

© 2009 Jack A. Apsche, EdD, ABPP

Scoring and Interpretation of the CCBQ-S

Results of the CCBQ-S identify life-threatening and life-interfering beliefs, as well as types of personality beliefs in the adolescent. The worksheets provided in the following pages guide you through the scoring and interpretation process. But first, let us take a closer look at life-threatening and treatment-interfering beliefs.

Life-Threatening and Treatment-Interfering Beliefs

As previously discussed in this chapter, life-threatening beliefs have associations with suicidal, parasuicidal, and other at-risk behaviors; while treatment-interfering beliefs are associated with avoidant behaviors. Life-threatening beliefs are identified in the following items on the CCBQ-S: 12, 21, 31, 32, 38, 43, 61, 73, 80. Treatment Interfering Beliefs are identified in the following items: 1, 4, 13, 17, 23, 24, 30, 39, 41, 56, 58, 66, 74, 84, 85, 87, 91. Both types of beliefs often help activate and trigger the modes, common to T1 and T2 (explained in chapter 8), as well as the fear and avoidance reaction (discussed in chapter 7) in the adolescent. These beliefs should be reviewed as a priority for the development of the Conglomerate of Beliefs and Behaviors, and the Triggers, Fears, Avoids, Compound Core Beliefs Correlation (chapter 8), as well as for the development of the Case Conceptualization (chapter 7).

When scoring life-threatening beliefs, "Always" (4), "Almost Always" (3) and "Sometimes" (2) responses are noted. Although "3" and "4" responses present a more severe profile of beliefs, due to the danger of the at-risk behavior identified in life-threatening beliefs, the clinician needs to also take into consideration "2" responses. On the CCBQ-S, check the box marked LT (Life-Threatening) for questions with "4," "3," or "2" responses. Then transfer these responses to the Life-Threatening and Treatment-Interfering Beliefs Worksheet on the next page. Follow the same procedure to score the treatment-interfering beliefs. First, on the CCBQ-S, place a check in the box marked TI (Treatment-Interfering) for items with "4" or "3" responses. Then, transfer these responses to the Life-Threatening and Treatment-Interfering Beliefs Worksheet. Take your time and review the results in order to identify patterns or clusters of beliefs in the adolescent and determine critical areas that may need to be addressed first in MDT treatment.

MDT CCBQ-S Life-Threatening and Treatment-Interfering Beliefs Worksheet

Name: _____ Date: _____

Life-Threatening Beliefs

Circle the 4 (Always), 3 (Almost Always), or 2 (Sometimes) level responses obtained in the CCBQ-S to the items below.

Item	Always	Almost Always	Sometimes	Item	Always	Almost Always	Sometimes
12	4	3	2	43	4	3	2
21	4	3	2	61	4	3	2
31	4	3	2	73	4	3	2
32	4	3	2	80	4	3	2
38	4	3	2				

Treatment-Interfering Beliefs

Circle the 3 (Almost Always) or 4 (Always) level responses obtained in the CCBQ-S to the items below.

Item	Always	Almost Always	Item	Always	Almost Always	Item	Always	Almost Always
1	4	3	30	4	3	74	4	3
4	4	3	39	4	3	84	4	3
13	4	3	41	4	3	85	4	3
17	4	3	56	4	3	87	4	3
23	4	3	58	4	3	91	4	3
24	4	3	66	4	3			

Types of Personality Beliefs

As previously indicated, the 96 items in the CCBQ-S are divided into eight types of beliefs (I–VIII). Each type includes 12 items and correlates with a specific personality belief or trait. The Roman numeral found at the end of each item of the CCBQ-S identifies the type of belief for that particular item. The types of beliefs and the items in which they are found are listed below.

I. Antisocial Personality Beliefs	Items: 8, 13, 39, 40, 42, 49, 55, 58, 63, 66, 74, 81
II. Avoidant Personality Beliefs	Items: 7, 12, 23, 26, 32, 35, 38, 44, 45, 53, 56, 61
III. Borderline Personality Beliefs	Items: 1, 5, 10, 21, 25, 27, 31, 37, 43, 46, 47, 50
IV. Conduct Beliefs	Items: 2, 6, 11, 22, 60, 68, 72, 73, 75, 77, 80, 82
V. Dependent Personality Beliefs	Items: 3, 15, 19, 24, 28, 33, 52, 59, 67, 70, 71, 79
VI. Histrionic Personality Beliefs	Items: 14, 18, 51, 54, 57, 62, 64, 65, 69, 76, 78, 83
VII. Narcissistic Personality Beliefs	Items: 4, 9, 17, 20, 30, 34, 36, 41, 84, 88, 90, 94
VIII. Obsessive-Compulsive Beliefs	Items: 16, 29, 48, 85, 86, 87, 89, 91, 92, 93, 95, 96

To score the CCBQ-S, circle all beliefs endorsed on the assessment as 4 ("Always") and 3 ("Almost Always") on the Scoring Worksheet and Profile Chart provided on the next page. Then, proceed to the CCBQ-S Profile Chart. To complete the Profile Chart, provide the number of endorsed 4 ("Always") and 3 ("Almost Always") responses for each type of belief (I–VIII), adding them (3s + 4s) in the respective total column. Carefully review the completed chart—it provides a blueprint of the types of beliefs that are fueling the adolescent's behavior. Look at the grouping of beliefs to infer possible developing personality disorder traits in the adolescent.

MDT PROFILE CHART & CCBQ-S SCORING WORKSHEET

Profile Chart

Name: _____   Date: _____

Antisocial Personality Beliefs

Item	Always	Almost Always	Item	Always	Almost Always	Item	Always	Almost Always
8	4	3	42	4	3	63	4	3
13	4	3	49	4	3	66	4	3
39	4	3	55	4	3	74	4	3
40	4	3	58	4	3	81	4	3

Avoidant Personality Beliefs

Item	Always	Almost Always	Item	Always	Almost Always	Item	Always	Almost Always
7	4	3	32	4	3	45	4	3
12	4	3	35	4	3	53	4	3
23	4	3	38	4	3	56	4	3
26	4	3	44	4	3	61	4	3

Borderline Personality Beliefs

Item	Always	Almost Always	Item	Always	Almost Always	Item	Always	Almost Always
1	4	3	25	4	3	43	4	3
5	4	3	27	4	3	46	4	3
10	4	3	31	4	3	47	4	3
21	4	3	37	4	3	50	4	3

Conduct Beliefs

Item	Always	Almost Always	Item	Always	Almost Always	Item	Always	Almost Always
2	4	3	60	4	3	75	4	3
6	4	3	68	4	3	77	4	3

| 11 | 4 | 3 | 72 | 4 | 3 | 80 | 4 | 3 |
| 22 | 4 | 3 | 73 | 4 | 3 | 82 | 4 | 3 |

Dependent Personality Beliefs

Item	Always	Almost Always	Item	Always	Almost Always	Item	Always	Almost Always
3	4	3	28	4	3	67	4	3
15	4	3	33	4	3	70	4	3
19	4	3	52	4	3	71	4	3
24	4	3	59	4	3	79	4	3

Histrionic Personality Beliefs

Item	Always	Almost Always	Item	Always	Almost Always	Item	Always	Almost Always
14	4	3	57	4	3	69	4	3
18	4	3	62	4	3	76	4	3
51	4	3	64	4	3	78	4	3
54	4	3	65	4	3	83	4	3

Narcissistic Personality Beliefs

Item	Always	Almost Always	Item	Always	Almost Always	Item	Always	Almost Always
4	4	3	30	4	3	84	4	3
9	4	3	34	4	3	88	4	3
17	4	3	36	4	3	90	4	3
20	4	3	41	4	3	94	4	3

Obsessive-Compulsive Beliefs

Item	Always	Almost Always	Item	Always	Almost Always	Item	Always	Almost Always
16	4	3	86	4	3	92	4	3
29	4	3	87	4	3	93	4	3
48	4	3	89	4	3	95	4	3
85	4	3	91	4	3	96	4	3

© 2009 Jack A. Apsche, EdD, ABPP

CCBQ-S Scoring Worksheet

Name: _____ Date: _____

	Personality Beliefs	**# of 4s Endorsed**	**# of 3s Endorsed**	**Total (3s + 4s)**
I.	Antisocial Personality Beliefs			
II.	Avoidant Personality Beliefs			
III.	Borderline Personality Beliefs			
IV.	Conduct Beliefs			
V.	Dependent Personality Beliefs			
VI.	Histrionic Personality Beliefs			
VII.	Narcissistic Personality Beliefs			
VIII.	Obsessive-Compulsive Beliefs			

© 2009 Jack A. Apsche, EdD, ABPP

Summary

The MDT CCBQ-S helps identify the adolescent's underlying beliefs and thoughts that guide his/ her behavior. It also pinpoints life-threatening and treatment-interfering beliefs, as well as specific types of personality beliefs and traits important to address in MDT treatment. Let's review some CCBQ-S administration guidelines: review the assessment prior to administration and highlight beliefs endorsed by the adolescent's presenting behavior and/or history; clarify each belief and give examples; take your time to complete the assessment—use several sessions if necessary; complete the assessment together with the adolescent; and remember to explore why if the adolescent does not endorse a belief you highlighted. The next chapter introduces you to the MDT case conceptualization process.

Chapter 7

Introduction to the MDT Case Conceptualization

The case conceptualization guides the MDT therapeutic treatment plan. It is a comprehensive protocol the MDT clinician uses to develop a functional treatment methodology. Through the evolution of the case conceptualization, the clinician delves deeper into the adolescent's underlying fears and beliefs, which are at the crux of the youth's avoidant and problematic behavior(s), as well as the internalizing and externalizing disorders. By identifying these fears and beliefs and their accompanying behaviors, the clinician and the adolescent collaboratively forge a blueprint for the MDT intervention.

A thorough understanding of the case conceptualization is pivotal to MDT treatment; therefore, we have dedicated three chapters (including this one) to its review. In this chapter, we present an overview of the case conceptualization; first providing a blank case conceptualization, followed by a completed example, and then explaining steps I through III. Steps IV to VI of the case conceptualization are discussed in chapter 8, and steps VII and VIII are discussed in chapter 9. We intend for this presentation design to provide greater clarity, understanding, and confidence in the development and implementation of the MDT Case Conceptualization.

Case Conceptualization Overview

The Case Conceptualization encapsulates data gathered from the Typology Survey (chapter 4), the Reactive-Proactive Scale (chapter 4), the Fear Assessment (chapter 5), and the Compound Core Belief Questionnaire – S (chapter 6). It is a stepwise process composed of the following eight steps:

Step I: Relevant Childhood Data (Abuse History)

Step II: Behavioral Data

Step III: Diagnoses

Step IV: Triggers, Fears, Avoids, Compound Core Beliefs Correlation (TFAB)

Step V: Conglomerate of Beliefs and Behaviors (COBB)

Step VI: Situational Analysis

Step VII: Mode Activation/Deactivation

Step VIII: Functional Treatment Development Form (FTDF)

Steps I through III target the adolescent's background data. Steps IV to VI identify and correlate the fears, beliefs, and behaviors that drive the adolescent. Steps VII and VIII further evaluate the activation and deactivation of the adolescent's fears, beliefs, and behaviors, in order to create a viable functional treatment plan. We recommend that you complete each step sequentially, as each one builds upon the previous one. Take a moment now to review the next few pages and familiarize yourself with all of the steps in the case conceptualization before learning about each step in more detail.

MDT Case Conceptualization

Name: _____   Date: _____

Gender: _____

Step I: Relevant Childhood Data (Abuse History)

Date of Birth:
Physical/Emotional Abuse:
Sexual Abuse:
Developmental History:
Substance Abuse History:
Current Medication(s):

Step II: Behavioral Data

Step III: Diagnoses

Axis I
Axis II
Axis III
Axis IV
Axis V Current GAF Highest GAF Past Year

Step IV: Triggers, Fears, Avoids, Compound Core Beliefs Correlation (TFAB)

Trigger 1 Conscious Processing	Trigger 2 Unconscious Processing	Fear	Avoids	Compound Core Beliefs

Step V: Conglomerate of Beliefs and Behaviors (COBB)

Compound Core Belief	Corresponding Behavior(s)

Step VI: Situational Analysis

Situation 1		Situation 2		Situation 3
Trigger 1	FEAR	Trigger 1	FEAR	Trigger 1
Trigger 2		Trigger 2		Trigger 2
Activated Compound Core Belief		Activated Compound Core Belief		Activated Compound Core Belief

Physiological Response		Physiological Response		Physiological Response
Emotional Response		Emotional Response		Emotional Response
Behavior(s)		Behavior(s)		Behavior(s)

Step VII: Mode Activation/Deactivation

Orienting Schema – Event:	
Anticipated Event	Preconscious Processing:
Perception of Fear	Physiological System:
Activation	Meaning Assignments, Memories, Beliefs:
Affective Schema	Behavioral Schema:
Motivational Schema	Attack:
Avoid(s):	

Step VIII: Functional Treatment Development Form (FTDF)

Functional Alternative Belief(s)	Healthy Alternative Thoughts	Functional Alternative Compensatory Strategy	Functional Reinforcing Behavior(s)	Specific Functional Treatment (Individual Treatment to Environment)	Validation, Clarification, Redirection (VCR)

© 2009 Jack A. Apsche, EdD, ABPP

There are various ways of completing the Case Conceptualization. When administering it for the first time, we recommend you address each step separately; that is, complete the Triggers, Fears, Avoids, Compound Core Beliefs Correlation (step IV) and the Conglomerate of Beliefs and Behaviors (step V) with the adolescent during individual sessions and the other sections on your own without the youth. As you become more fluent in MDT, you can complete a greater number of the steps or components together with the adolescent until you feel adept at completing the entire case conceptualization collaboratively with the youth. A completed Case Conceptualization would look like the one below.

MDT Example Case Conceptualization

Step I: Relevant Childhood Data (Abuse History)

Date of Birth: 8/4/95
Physical/Emotional Abuse: *Physical abuse—victimized by neighborhood gangs. Neglected by mother and family.*
Sexual Abuse: *None*
Developmental History: *Fifteen years old (15). All developmental milestones appropriate. Has a younger brother, 8-years-old and a 4-year-old sister. His father has no contact with him and is currently incarcerated. History of frequent early childhood aggression.*
Substance Abuse History: *States he used marijuana, one to two blunts per day. Mother had an alcohol problem, in remission.*
Current Medication(s): *N/A*

Step II: Behavioral Data

1. *Incarcerated in juvenile facility for assault of teacher and peers.*

2. *Removed from home for truancy and assault of neighbor.*

Step III: Diagnoses

Axis I: *312.81 Conduct Disorder, Childhood Onset Type.*

312.30 Impulse Control Disorder NOS

Axis II: *Narcissistic traits*

Axis III: *Asthma*

Axis IV: *Psychosocial and legal problems*

Axis V: Current GAF: *35* Highest GAF Past Year: *34*

Step IV: Triggers, Fears, Avoids, Compound Core Beliefs Correlation (TFAB)

Trigger 1 Conscious Processing	Trigger 2 Unconscious Processing	Fear	Avoids	Compound Core Beliefs
I must protect myself.	*You will hurt me.*	*Fear of trusting anyone.*	*Closeness and intimacy.*	*Everyone betrays my trust, I cannot trust anyone.*
I must not feel.	*I am weak and vulnerable.*	*Fear something is wrong with me.*	*Intimacy/feelings/ emotional pain.*	*Whenever I feel, it will be unpleasant.*
I must be strong and powerful.	*I am weak.*	*Fear of never being real with my problems.*	*Being real.*	*Whenever I am angry, my emotions go from annoyed to furious.*
I can't let you see who I am.	*I am defective.*	*Fear someone will get me if I let my guard down.*	*Trust/closeness.*	*Other people's feelings are not as important as mine. If I don't take care of them first, they will get me.*

Step V: Conglomerate of Beliefs and Behaviors (COBB)

Compound Core Belief	Corresponding Behavior(s)
Everyone betrays my trust, I cannot trust anyone.	*Threaten, punch.*
Whenever I feel, it will be unpleasant.	*Shut down, isolate, aggression.*
Whenever I am angry, my emotions go from annoyed to furious.	*Physical and verbal aggression.*
Other people's feelings are not as important as mine. If I don't get them first, they will get me.	*Aggression.*

Step VI: Situational Analysis

Situation 1 *Got into an argument with peer and punched peer.*	FEAR	Situation 2 *Argument with mother in a family session.*	FEAR	Situation 3 *Is confronted by staff for being loud.*
Trigger 1 *I must protect myself.*		Trigger 1 *I must not feel.*		Trigger 1 *I must be strong.*
Trigger 2 *You will hurt me.*		Trigger 2 *I am weak.*		Trigger 2 *I am weak.*
Avoids *Trust*		Avoids *Feelings*		Avoids *Being real, looking weak*
Activated Compound Core Belief *If I don't get you first, you will get me.*		Activated Compound Core Belief *Whenever I feel, it is horrible.*		Activated Compound Core Belief *If I get disrespected, I blow up.*
Physiological Response *Breathing fast, clenched fists.*		Physiological Response *Numb*		Physiological Response *Tight jaw, heart pumping, clenched fists.*
Emotional Response *Anger*		Emotional Response *Numb*		Emotional Response *Numb*
Behavior(s) *Punch*		Behavior(s) *Isolate or run.*		Behavior(s) *Attack staff member.*

Step VII: Mode Activation/Deactivation

Orienting Schema – Event: *Meeting with school authority.*	
Anticipated Event: *"I must protect myself."*	Preconscious Processing: *"Others will hurt me."*
Perception of Fear: *Trust and mistrust.*	Physiological System: *Heart pounding, tight jaw.*
Activation: *Disrespect/condescension.*	Meaning Assignments, Memories, Beliefs: *"Everyone betrays my trust."*
Affective Schema: *Numb*	Behavioral Schema: *Aggression.*
Motivational Schema: *Protect self.*	Attack: *Remove threat by anger and aggression.*
Avoid(s): *Isolation.*	

Step VIII: Functional Treatment Development Form (FTDF)

Functional Alternative Belief	Healthy Alternative Thoughts	Functional Alternative Compensatory Strategy	Functional Reinforcing Behaviors	Specific Functional Treatment (Individual Treatment to Environment)	Validation, Clarification, Redirection (VCR)
I can trust people sometimes.	I will take a small step at a time with trust.	Mindfulness, breathing, MDT skill set.	Use trust scale situational.	Mindfulness, trust scales.	V: You make sense not to trust people given your life experiences. C: It seems, though, that we have been honest with each other thus far in our relationship, so in this right here and now…. R: Is it possible that you can, in this moment, trust me a little, say on a scale of 1 to 10?
At times, I can feel and it will be okay.	I will allow myself to defuse my feelings in therapy.	Mindfulness, acceptance, defusion of painful feelings.	Experience feelings in a safe place (therapy).	Mindfulness, acceptance with one staff worker I trust.	V: You have lived your life avoiding feelings because of not wanting to experience the pain. I understand that fully. C: But you may want to consider experiencing the feelings and moving forward without avoiding the fear of feeling. R: But at this moment you experienced feelings okay for a brief second. Is it possible for you to feel and it is okay?
I can deal with my anger sometimes.	I can see what other people want.	MDT mindfulness treatment.	Measure how important their feelings are on a scale of 1 to 10.	Mindfulness, breathing, evaluate other's needs.	V: I understand why you get so angry and aggressive. You have been beaten up and abused your whole life. C: But you, here at times, have been able to interrupt your anger and aggression by breathing and mindfulness. R: Is it possible for you to practice your MDT breathing skills and use MDT mindfulness skill set now, on a scale of 1 to 10?

Functional Alternative Belief	Healthy Alternative Thoughts	Functional Alternative Compensatory Strategy	Functional Reinforcing Behaviors	Specific Functional Treatment (Individual Treatment to Environment)	Validation, Clarification, Redirection (VCR)
Others' feelings might be important sometimes.	I will breathe and separate myself from my anger and aggression.	Breathing, mindfulness of self.	Step back and breathe, take a break from anger.	Mindfulness, MDT breathing.	V: It makes sense why you have to worry about yourself first and not others. C: But you might be able to see others' feelings sometimes. You mentioned that you worry about your brother. R: So is it possible that you might be able to consider his feelings as important as yours right here in the moment?
At times, I don't have to punch others over a disagreement.	I can step back and see what this person really wants.	Step back, breathe, and listen.	Measure my risk 1 to 10.	Ask for help if mediation with a peer is still necessary.	V: It makes sense why you feel you have to hurt others. You had your butt kicked by others when you were young. C: But it just got you in trouble with the law, so do you think it might not be a good thing at the moment? R: Is it possible you could check out the situation and trust yourself in the moment not to have "to kill them all and let God sort it out"? Just in the moment, right here and now?

© 2009 Jack A. Apsche, EdD, ABPP

Throughout the completion of the case conceptualization, it is important to be aware of additional behavioral and emotional clues that can help you gain greater insight about the adolescent. Now that you have seen an example of a completed case conceptualization, let's explore the pathway to complete learning the process. Using the example of the adolescent provided above, we begin by taking a closer look at the first three steps: step I, Relevant Childhood Data (Abuse History); step II, Behavioral Data; and step III, Diagnoses. As indicated at the beginning of this chapter, steps I to III of the case conceptualization capture the adolescent's background data.

Step I: Relevant Childhood Data (Abuse History)

The first step in the case conceptualization refers to childhood information about the adolescent. You have already obtained the majority of this information in the Typology Survey. Having to sift through the data in order to obtain the necessary information for the case conceptualization comes with a potential benefit of reviewing it from a different perspective and perhaps noticing significant items you initially overlooked. If you find that you do not have all of the information needed, you can obtain it from the adolescent or a collateral source such as the parent/guardian, from files, or by other means. Besides identifying information such as date of birth, data recorded in step I includes Physical/Emotional Abuse, Sexual Abuse, Developmental History, Substance Abuse, and Medications. We record the adolescent's abuse history—physical, emotional, and sexual—because there is a correlation between these traumatic childhood experiences and the subsequent development of internalizing and externalizing disorders. The developmental section captures behavioral, environmental, social, and biological information. Developmental milestones are recorded and, of particular importance, it is the behavioral component of this section where you review the adolescent's history of self- and other-inflicted aggression. That is, you report any past known other aggression such as verbal and physical altercations, destruction of property, gang activity, criminal history, sex offending behavior, and so on. The youth's history of self-aggression (or self-harm), such as cutting, parasuicide, and suicidal behaviors, is also recorded. Any familial or environmental factors deemed influential in the development of the youth's problematic behaviors are included. If there is chemical dependence, note the drug of choice, frequency of use, familial substance abuse history, and any other pertinent information. Lastly, for data on prescribed medications, complete step I of the Case Conceptualization as shown in the example below.

Date of Birth: 8/4/95
Physical/Emotional Abuse: *Physical abuse - victimized by neighborhood gangs. Neglected by mother and family.*
Sexual Abuse: *None*

Developmental History: *Fifteen years old (15). All developmental milestones appropriate. Has a younger brother, 8-years-old and a 4-year-old sister. His father has no contact with him and is currently incarcerated. History of frequent early childhood aggression.*	
Substance Abuse History: *States he used marijuana, one to two blunts per day. Mother had an alcohol problem, in remission.*	
Current Medication(s): *N/A*	

Step II: Behavioral Data

This section differs from the developmental behavioral data in step I in that here (step II) you record the adolescent's more current behavioral problems. You also include results obtained from assessments such as the Youth Self Report or the Child Behavior Checklist, as well as relevant information from the Typology Survey. A completed step II might look like this:

1. *Incarcerated in juvenile facility for assault of teacher and peers.*

2. *Removed from home for truancy and assault of a neighbor.*

Step III: Diagnoses

If the adolescent has been formally diagnosed, include the information in this section. The results of the CCBQ-S (chapter 6), based on the beliefs endorsed by the adolescent, should be congruent with any Axis II diagnoses.

Axis I	*312.81 Conduct Disorder, Childhood Onset Type* *312.30 Impulse Control Disorder*
Axis II	*Narcissistic traits*
Axis III	*Asthma*
Axis IV	*Psychosocial and legal problems*
Axis V	*Current GAF: 35* *Highest GAF Past Year: 34*

Take a moment to review the first three steps of the Case Conceptualization. It deepens your understanding of the adolescent, as well as provides a solid base for the next steps.

Summary

This chapter introduced you to the MDT case conceptualization. It is a systematic and thoughtful process designed to gather a vast amount of information about the adolescent. As you can see, it is also an elaborate process in which each step builds upon the preceding one. Take your time as you familiarize yourself with the case conceptualization. Review the completed example. When you feel that you have mastered steps I through III, move forward to the next chapter. Chapter 8 focuses on developing collaboration with the adolescent in order to complete steps IV through VI.

Chapter 8

Developing Treatment and Collaboration

In this chapter we continue describing the case conceptualization, specifically step IV, Triggers, Fears, Avoids, Compound Core Beliefs Correlation (TFAB); step V, Conglomerate of Beliefs and Behaviors (COBB); and step VI, Situational Analysis. These steps represent a much deeper collaborative alliance between the clinician and the adolescent. For the youth, it is the process of explaining the beliefs endorsed in the MDT Fear Assessment and the CCBQ-S. At this stage of MDT, the adolescent has the opportunity to verbalize personal primary beliefs in a safe environment and in his/her own words. It is a vulnerable stand for the adolescent, so the clinician needs to take care that the youth does not feel threatened, judged, or belittled. The clinician encourages the youth's disclosures and participation through acceptance and validation of the adolescent's grain of truth; that is, acceptance and validation that what the youth experiences at a particular moment is his/her reality and, thus, belief in life. The clinician then guides the adolescent in discovering correlations between past experiences, beliefs, and behaviors through the steps in the MDT case conceptualization. Step IV, discussed next, begins this journey.

Step IV: Triggers, Fears, Avoids, Compound Core Beliefs Correlation

The Triggers, Fears, Avoids, Compound Core Beliefs Correlation (TFAB) delineates a concrete correlation between all the elements in its name: triggers → fears → avoids → compound core beliefs. In fact, this sequence represents the actual chain reaction from triggers to beliefs in the adolescent that precedes problematic behavior and/or internalizing disorders. However, in order to uncover the reason for the activation and source of a belief, we begin by identifying the particular belief first and work backward through the chain until reaching the instigating factor (trigger). Therefore, the TFAB is completed from right to left (compound core beliefs → avoids →

fears → triggers), which explains why we begin our discussion with the Compound Core Beliefs (far right column).

Compound Core Beliefs

Compound core beliefs refer to those underlying beliefs that, as explained in chapter 6, can lead to the development of particular life-threatening and treatment-interfering beliefs in the adolescent. To complete the Compound Core Beliefs column of the TFAB, you refer to the beliefs already endorsed on the Compound Core Beliefs Questionnaire – S. As previously explained, these beliefs are at the crux of the adolescent's unhealthy or problematic behavior and develop as a result of the youth's past experiences (underlying beliefs). When self-integrated into the adolescent's belief system, underlying beliefs influence the youth's overall life perceptions and reactions. Furthermore, underlying beliefs may lead the adolescent to engage in high-risk behaviors (life-threatening beliefs) or may strengthen avoidant behaviors detrimental to therapeutic interventions (treatment-interfering beliefs). Compound core beliefs are also used when completing step V, Conglomerate of Beliefs and Behaviors (COBB), of the case conceptualization. The clinician and the adolescent collaboratively complete the Compound Core Beliefs column through reviewing the beliefs endorsed in the CCBQ-S. Throughout the discussion, the clinician accepts and validates the youth's perception of his/her reality in order to encourage and support honest participation in this exercise. The TFAB at this point would look like this:

Trigger 1 Conscious Processing	Trigger 2 Unconscious Processing	Fear	Avoids	Compound Core Beliefs
				Everyone betrays my trust, I cannot trust anyone.

The clinician and the adolescent are now ready to proceed to the next column: Avoids. However, the Avoids are actually part of the Fear → Avoids paradigm, explained below.

The Fear-Avoids Paradigm

The Fear → Avoids paradigm illustrates the direct correlation between what the adolescent fears and what he/she avoids; this can also be expressed as what the adolescent avoids comes from what he/she fears. Although we discuss the avoids and the fears separately for the purpose of explaining how to complete the TFAB, please understand that they are sometimes so interwoven in their presentation that they may be hard to discern from each other, requiring careful evaluation and discussion between you and the adolescent.

AVOIDS

As previously explained, avoids originate from fear(s). They can serve as coping mechanisms or nonfunctional alternatives to fears. However, similar to the fight and flight response, their overuse may create an unhealthy or dysfunctional pattern to life's events. Furthermore, avoids mask the core of vulnerability in the adolescent while simultaneously increasing this self-perceived weakness in the youth. For example, if the adolescent fears betrayal by others, he/she may avoid having a best friend; or, if the adolescent fears being the center of attention, he/she may avoid public speaking situations.

We have identified a few typical patterns of avoids and their corresponding originating fears. By listing them here, we do not imply that their coupling is absolute for all adolescents. In other words, these fears may result in these avoids or these avoids may be a result of these fears. Each adolescent comes with a unique history of experiences, perceptions, and interpretations, and the clinician needs to respect and understand that individuality. Thus, we provide the following fear → avoids examples as a starting point for you and the adolescent to evaluate some of his/her avoids, in order to identify the particular fear(s) that may fuel the youth's avoidant behavior(s).

Fear → Avoids

- *Failing* → *Trying new behaviors*

- *Anger* → *Confrontation, being a victim*

- *Feelings* → *Close relationships*

- *Trust* → *Relationship*

- *Being different* → *Being honest*

You can see that to successfully identify the avoids, you also may need to concurrently identify the fears that fuel the youth. Remember that these are extremely vulnerable areas in many adolescents, so proceed with care, acceptance, and validation; and refrain from judging a fear or avoids.

FEARS

The results from the Fear Assessment presented in chapter 5 can help you complete the Fear column of the TFAB. To briefly review, the Fear Assessment provides a venue for identifying fears that result from underlying anxieties that fuel experiential avoidance and dysfunctional behaviors in adolescents. The Life-Interfering Fears Worksheet of the Fear Assessment pinpoints 21 fears that are often the source of unhealthy behaviors in adolescents. Additionally, the five subcategories in the Fear Assessment (Personal Reactive–External Index, Personal Reactive–Internal/ Self-Concept Index, Environmental Index, Physical Index, and Abuse Index) examine different fear reactions in the adolescent. The Personal Reactive–External Index, in particular, identifies internal fears reactive to external events. These fears originate from past negative experiences and serve as triggers for the cognitive conscious (T1) and subconscious (T2) that activate aggressive and oppositional behaviors in the adolescent. They are activated by external stimuli and generate the highest level of anxiety in the adolescent. Although all fears endorsed by the adolescent are important, the life-interfering fears and the Personal Reactive–External fears are of greater concern, clinically. You can use the completed Fear Assessment as the springboard to collaboratively complete the Fear column of the TFAB with the adolescent. Start with the fear or the avoids, whichever is easier for the adolescent; one will lead to the other. At this stage, your TFAB would look like this:

Trigger 1 Conscious Processing	Trigger 2	Unconscious Processing	Fear	Avoids	Compound Core Beliefs
			Fear of trusting anyone.	*Closeness and intimacy.*	*Everyone betrays my trust, I cannot trust anyone.*

The Fear → Avoids paradigm is also significantly related to Triggers 1 and 2, discussed next.

Triggers

The fear, avoidance, and compound core beliefs are activated by triggers specific to the adolescent. In other words, depending on the adolescent's past experiences and perceptions, a person, an object, a sound, a touch, a smell, or other stimuli can activate the fear → avoid paradigm, in turn, arousing unhealthy beliefs (compound core beliefs).

In MDT, we make the distinction between two types of triggers: Trigger 1 (T1) and Trigger 2 (T2). T1s are closely related to the fears listed in the TFAB and are part of the adolescent's conscious processing; that is, the adolescent is aware of these fears. T2s, on the other hand, constitute the unconscious processing—in other words, the adolescent is unaware of having these fears but they still result in behavior(s) observable by others. T2s are the reason for the avoids listed in the TFAB. Sometimes, however, a trigger can have both dimensions, conscious and unconscious processing. Let's review how the TFAB would look at this point before further explanation of T1s and T2s.

Trigger 1 Conscious Processing	Trigger 2 Unconscious Processing	Fear	Avoids	Compound Core Beliefs
I must protect myself.	*You will hurt me.*	*Fear of trusting anyone.*	*Closeness and intimacy.*	*Everyone betrays my trust, I cannot trust anyone.*

In the example above, T1, "I must protect myself," activates the "Fear of trusting anyone," while T2, "You will hurt me," activates the avoidance of "Closeness and intimacy." The triggers, fear, and avoids, in turn, activate the compound core belief "Everyone betrays my trust, I cannot trust anyone." This chain of reactions in the adolescent results in unhealthy and dysfunctional behavior. The TFAB crystallizes the relationship between all of its components so that both the adolescent and the clinician can better grasp what fuels the oppositional, angry, or aggressive adolescent. After completing the TFAB, we also like the adolescent to complete the Client TFAB Collaborative Worksheet. Through this worksheet, the youth verbalizes in his/her own words the beliefs endorsed in previous MDT assessments, as well as relates these beliefs to his/her behaviors. Here's an example of how a clinician can work with the youth to complete the TFAB Collaborative Worksheet.

Therapist: Let's take a look at some of the beliefs that you endorsed in the CCBQ-S, okay?

Adolescent: Sure, what are we doing with them?

Therapist: I would like to see if we can get you to put them in your words so they mean something to you.

Adolescent: I can do that.

Therapist: How would you word, "Everyone betrays my trust, I cannot trust anyone."

Adolescent: I can't trust anyone unless I know them, and they still may screw me.

Therapist: Of your friends, how many do you think will screw you?

Adolescent: Maybe 90 percent of my friends will still screw me over.

Therapist: So maybe like this, "I can't trust anyone unless I get to know them. They will not hurt me 10 percent of the time."

Adolescent: Yeah, that sounds right.

Therapist: That is good, how about another belief?

Adolescent: Yeah, okay.

Therapist: Now, how about this belief, "Whenever I feel, it will be unpleasant."

Adolescent: I don't like to feel.

Therapist: Can you tell me why?

Adolescent: Feeling makes me soft and weak.

Therapist: Okay, why is that?

Adolescent: 'Cause feelings make you weak and you can get hurt where I am from.

Therapist: Okay, good. I don't like to feel, it makes me weak.

Adolescent: Yeah, that's it.

Therapist: Great work…let's keep this going.

A completed example of the Client TFAB Collaborative Worksheet is provided below. You will notice that the worksheet has two additional columns to the right of the columns already listed in the TFAB: My Belief System and My Behaviors.

Client TFAB Collaborative Worksheet

Trigger 1 Conscious Processing	Trigger 2 Unconscious Processing	Fear	Avoids	Compound Core Beliefs	My Belief System	My Behaviors
I must protect myself.	*You will hurt me.*	*Fear of trusting anyone.*	*Closeness and intimacy.*	*Everyone betrays my trust, I cannot trust anyone.*	*I can't trust anyone unless I know them. Then 90% of the time they will hurt me.*	*If I don't trust you, I will threaten or punch you.*

The Client TFAB Collaborative Worksheet prepares the clinician and the adolescent for the next step in the case conceptualization: step V, Conglomerate of Beliefs and Behaviors.

Step V: Conglomerate of Beliefs and Behaviors

The Conglomerate of Beliefs and Behaviors (COBB) synthesizes the beliefs and behaviors identified in the CCBQ-S and in the TFAB. In the CCBQ-S, the adolescent endorsed the beliefs; in the TFAB he/she evaluated the triggers, fears, and avoids that fuel those beliefs; and in the Client TFAB Collaborative Worksheet, the youth translated the endorsed beliefs into his/her own words and acknowledged the accompanying behavior(s). Through this sequential process, the youth gains awareness of the correlation between particular beliefs and his/her emotional and behavioral dysregulation. In the COBB, the adolescent further correlates unhealthy beliefs with their specific accompanying unhealthy behaviors in order to be able to (in the future) balance beliefs as a pathway to emotional and behavioral self-regulation. Acceptance and validation by the adolescent and the clinician of the compound core beliefs and the corresponding behaviors are central to the COBB.

Completing the COBB is a collaborative exercise between the client and the clinician and is the basis for the treatment hypothesis. The completed COBB becomes a living document integral to the adolescent's therapeutic treatment. It transcends the clinician's office and is also used in collaboration with the youth's parents or caregivers. Acceptance of the COBB by the adolescent is a concrete demonstration of his/her commitment to treatment and behavioral change. The COBB also provides the clinician an avenue to further discern present and/or emerging personality beliefs and traits in the adolescent. These personality beliefs, particularly when presenting as clusters, can constitute obstinate treatment-interfering behaviors, meriting careful evaluation.

To begin to collaboratively complete the COBB with the adolescent, refer to the CCBQ-S and the Client TFAB Collaborative Worksheet. Encourage the youth to translate endorsed beliefs into his/her own words. For example, say to the adolescent, "Tell me in your own words what you mean by 'Whenever I hope, I will become disappointed.'" With some adolescents, you may have to provide your own paraphrasing of beliefs and then ask for confirmation from the youth that your rewording is accurate. For example, say to the youth, "When you endorsed the belief, 'Whenever I am angry, my emotions are extreme and out of control,' did you mean that, 'When you piss me off, I will go off and I can't control it?'" After you have identified the beliefs in the COBB with the adolescent, proceed to determine the accompanying behavior(s). For example, ask the adolescent, "What do you do when you believe that you cannot trust someone?" Make sure the adolescent specifies the resulting behavior for the belief. The COBB might look like the following example.

Compound Core Belief	Corresponding Behavior(s)
Everyone betrays my trust, I cannot trust anyone.	*Threaten, punch.*

Although the completed COBB would include additional beliefs and corresponding behavior(s), you may not be able to record all of the adolescent's beliefs. Therefore, you will need to prioritize the responses to ascertain that you address those beliefs that fuel the more severe aberrant behaviors in the youth and require immediate attention. These beliefs and behaviors are activated in particular contexts as presented in step VI: Situational Analysis.

Step VI: Situational Analysis

The Situational Analysis section of the Case Conceptualization evaluates the external environment or context in which the adolescent's behaviors occur. There are eight components to the Situational Analysis: Situation, Trigger 1, Trigger 2, Avoids, Activated Compound Core Belief, Physiological Response, Emotional Response, and Behaviors. Even though you are already familiar with some of these elements, let's look at each one briefly.

- **Situation** refers to the specific situation or event in which the behavior occurs.

- **Trigger 1** refers to the conscious thought or awareness that sets in motion the precursors to the behavior.

- **Trigger 2** refers to the unconscious or out-of-awareness processing that sets in motion the precursors to the behavior.

- **Avoids** refers to the reaction to the fear.

- **Activated Compound Core Belief** refers to the reaction to the fear. Remember, the fear activates the beliefs.

- **Physiological Response** refers to the ranked order of the physiological response.

- **Emotional Response** refers to the feelings present during the behavior.

- **Behaviors** refer to the actions presented in the identified situation.

We suggest that you include three different situations when completing the Situational Analysis. Completing multiple scenarios allows both the clinician and the youth to identify patterns in the youth's life. Let's look at what a completed column of a Situational Analysis might look like.

Situation 1 *Got into an argument with peer and punched peer.*
Trigger 1 *I must protect myself.*
Trigger 2 *You will hurt me.*
Avoids *Trust*
Activated Compound Core Belief *If I don't get you first, you will get me.*
Physiological Response *Breathing fast, clenched fists.*
Emotional Response *Anger*
Behavior(s) *Punch*

Step VI of the Case Conceptualization, the Situational Analysis, is a powerful exercise in which the adolescent identifies each step in the escalation and dysregulation of his/her reactions to particular events. The ability to understand the relationship between reactions and events is an empowering skill that moves the adolescent closer to gaining healthier self-control.

Summary

This chapter was essential in developing an understanding of how the collaborative process helps get the adolescent to "buy into" MDT. Honest clinician/adolescent collaboration requires that the clinician have a clear understanding of and be comfortable with the methodology. This strategy includes careful and active listening while engaging the adolescent in each step of the case conceptualization. It is essential that the youth translate personal beliefs into his/her own words. You will find that the adolescent is easy to engage in MDT as long as he/she understands the purpose of the case conceptualization and the collaborative process. Once you have practiced and mastered steps IV to VI in the development of the case conceptualization, you are prepared to address the function of the adolescent's problems, discussed in the next chapter.

Chapter 9

Functional Treatment Development Form

This chapter guides you through the two final steps of the MDT case conceptualization: Mode Activation/Deactivation (step VII) and Functional Treatment Development Form (step VIII). In chapter 2, we discussed how MDT is based on Beck's (1996) theoretical constructs of how modes provide the individual with alternative strategies to solve problems. We have found that oppositional, angry, and aggressive adolescents subscribe to an activation of unhealthy modes that guide their problematic behaviors. Consequently, the goal of MDT is to teach the adolescent to recognize the process of this detrimental mode activation and its consequences, and to empower the youth to deactivate an active mode appropriately in order to prevent engaging in unhealthy behaviors. Subsequently, after integrating mode deactivation into his/her personal schema, the adolescent learns how to replace the previous dysfunctional behaviors with alternative, healthier behaviors. Throughout this process, the youth gains greater emotional and behavioral self-control. Step VII of the case conceptualization graphically captures the adolescent's mode activation and subsequent mode deactivation.

Step VII: Mode Activation Deactivation

To understand mode deactivation, we need to first have a clear concept of mode activation. The following components are involved in this process: orienting schema, event, anticipated event, preconscious processing, perception, physiological system, activation, meaning assignments, memories, and beliefs, affective schema, behavioral schema, attack, and avoids. The following is a brief description of each of these elements involved in the mode activation process (Apsche, 2010).

- The **orienting schema** is the actual danger, fear, threat, signal, or charge experienced by the adolescent.

- The **event** is the actual situation that takes place that produces the fear experienced by the adolescent.

- The **anticipated event** is the adolescent's unconscious process of anticipation of a fear-evoking event.

- The **preconscious processing** is the adolescent's cognitive unconscious based on the experiences of danger-charged fears.

- The **perception of fear** is the adolescent's sense of fear that fully charges the mode activation system.

- The **physiological system** is the adolescent's network of physical responses to fear, arousal, or charges.

- The **activation** is the adolescent's cognitive schema(s) processing of fear-evoked beliefs or thoughts.

- The **meaning assignments, memories, and beliefs** are the adolescent's activation of the compound core beliefs.

- The **affective schema** is the adolescent's emotional component.

- The **behavioral schema** is the adolescent's behavior response to the activated belief.

- The **motivation schema** is the adolescent's alerting signal of the increasing need to escape the fear.

- The **attack** is the adolescent's response to eliminate the threat by aggression.

- The **avoid(s)** is the adolescent's response and/or escape from the fear in a noncontact form.

As you can see, the adolescent's mode activation is a complex process and thus merits careful evaluation. To complicate matters further, although we isolate the components in order to discuss each one, they often overlap with each other and occur concurrently, making it difficult (but not impossible) to determine their primacy or order of presentation. How does an adolescent's unhealthy mode activation appear in real time? Let's look at an adaptation of a case study to understand the actual MDT process.

• *Case Study: Mode Activation*

D. is a reactive adolescent in MDT treatment. He has a conglomerate of personality traits to suggest he endorsed multiple borderline personality beliefs on the CCBQ-S. He has a history of severe physical abuse, perceives threats in many situations, and feels threatened by authority figures. As D. perceives danger in a variety of situations, he reacts to prevent revictimization.

If D. perceives that he could be in a situation where there is a chance that he would be confronted or reprimanded, he would feel his anxiety increase. He can be involved in normal activities with a friend or peer, yet, if he notices the time getting closer to a group or meeting with "authority figures," he feels his anxiety increasing. Even if he is not increasingly thinking about the meeting, group, etc., some kind of preconscious processing of the anticipated event is occurring and producing anxiety. The knowledge that he will be involved in a situation that he perceives as a confrontation has already set in motion cognitive, affective, behavioral, and physiological processes.

As he draws closer to the time of the perceived/feared group or meeting, D. has a conscious fear or threat of being a victim. He feels his heart pounding and his chest tighten. He is fearful of becoming verbally and/or physically aggressive in order to protect himself. He thinks that he must protect himself. He can feel the pain turn to numbness in his chest. The situation presents a threat, real or perceived, based on his life experiences. D. feels both fearful of his own actions in this situation and later humiliated by the circumstances that surround the situation. He moves to punish the source of his fear and humiliation by punching the source of his perceived fear. He aggressed the source of his fear violently.

Analysis of Mode Activation

Let's look at the example presented above again, but this time with each of the mode activation components identified.

D. is a reactive adolescent in MDT treatment. He has a conglomerate of personality traits to suggest he endorsed multiple borderline personality beliefs on the CCBQ-S. He has a history of severe physical abuse, perceives threats in many situations, and feels threatened by authority figures. As D. perceives danger in a variety of situations, he reacts to prevent revictimization.

If D. perceives that he could be in a situation where there is a chance that he would be confronted or reprimanded, he would feel his anxiety increase (orienting schema). He can be involved in normal activities with a friend or peer, yet, if he notices the time getting closer to a group or meeting with "authority figures," he feels his anxiety increasing (event). Even if he is not increasingly thinking about the meeting (anticipated event), group, etc., some kind of preconscious processing of the anticipated event is occurring and producing anxiety (preconscious event). The knowledge that he will be involved in a situation (perception) that he perceives as a confrontation has already set in motion cognitive, affective, behavioral, and physiological processes.

As he draws closer to the time of the perceived/feared group or meeting, D. has a conscious fear or threat of being a victim (activation). He feels his heart pounding and his chest tighten (physiological system). He is fearful of becoming verbally and/or physically aggressive in order to protect himself. He thinks that he must protect himself (meaning assignments, memories, beliefs). He can feel the pain turn to numbness in his chest (affective schema). The situation presents a threat, real or perceived, based on his life experiences. D. feels both fearful of his own actions in this situation and later humiliated by the circumstances that surround the situation. He moves to punish the source of his fear and humiliation by punching the source of his perceived fear (behavioral schema). He aggressed the source of his fear violently (attack).

Now that you know how a mode is activated, let's explore how it can be deactivated.

Mode Deactivation

Imagine a female adolescent with escalating anxiety (fear) due to an upcoming case review with potential foster parents. Her T1, "You will hurt me," and T2, "I must protect myself," are already triggered and focused on her trust issues and her experience of being let down by many people in authority. Physiologically, she presents shallow breathing, clenched jaw, and closed fists. The activated belief is: "Everyone tells me one thing and does something different." Can you name the elements activated in her mode? The first step for the MDT clinician to teach this adolescent how to deactivate her mode prior to violence or other aberrant behaviors is to identify with the adolescent what and how her mode activates. The next step is to implement MDT treatment: mindfulness, emotional defusion, cognitive defusion, acceptance, and validation, clarification, and redirection of the adolescent's functional alternative belief. Mindfulness is the first step to decreasing the fear or negative perception of an event, as well as any physiological reaction accompanying prospective mode activators. Through MDT, the adolescent becomes fully aware of her difficulties with fear-invoking situations and typical physiological responses to this fear. Subsequently, she implements mindfulness and acceptance (chapter 11) to deactivate the mode. The aggressive response is then replaced by the steps in MDT treatment. The goal is to deactivate the adolescent's fear reaction to stimuli and reduce her experiential avoidance that many times manifests itself in oppositional, angry, and aggressive behaviors.

Understanding the mode activation and mode deactivation process in the adolescent allows the clinician to more effectively and accurately shape the youth's treatment hypothesis in the Functional Treatment Development Form (FTDF), the last step of the case conceptualization.

Step VIII: Functional Treatment Development Form

The final step to the MDT case conceptualization is the Functional Treatment Development Form (FTDF). As previously indicated, the FTDF outlines the treatment hypothesis and includes measurable therapeutic goals as well as experiential strategies. Its development is possible through the careful evaluation of the data gathered via the MDT methodology: Reactive–Proactive Scale, Typology Survey, Fear Assessment, Compound Core Belief Questionnaire (CCBQ-S), steps I–VII of the case conceptualization, and the collaborative relationship with the adolescent. The FTDF consists of six areas (columns), which combined, represent the adolescent's new (healthier) belief system; or rather, the belief system that the adolescent strives to integrate and implement through MDT therapy. These areas include: functional alternative belief(s); healthy alternative thought(s); functional alternative compensatory strategy; functional reinforcing behavior(s); specific functional treatment individual treatment to environment; and validation, clarification, and redirection.

Functional Alternative Beliefs

Let's begin with the first column, Functional Alternative Belief(s). These beliefs represent, first, the functional or healthy alternative to the life-interfering beliefs and, second, the treatment-interfering beliefs originally endorsed by the adolescent. To develop the functional alternative belief(s), review with the adolescent the compound core beliefs identified on the COBB. Explain to him/her that the compound core beliefs and the functional alternative beliefs are opposite to each other (to a degree). For example, if the compound core belief is "Everyone betrays my trust, I cannot trust anyone" then the functional alternative belief may be "I can trust people sometimes." You can see that the functional alternative belief moves the adolescent from the absolute stand of "no trust" to the position of the "possibility of trust." This shift in perspective provides the opportunity for viable incremental change through the acceptance of alternative beliefs, while allowing the adolescent to hold on to some of the past beliefs; thus, the process is less threatening for the youth. At this point the FTDF would look like this:

Functional Alternative Belief(s)	Healthy Alternative Thoughts	Functional Alternative Compensatory Strategy	Functional Reinforcing Behavior(s)	Specific Functional Treatment (Individual Treatment to Environment)	Validation, Clarification, Redirection (VCR)
I can trust people sometimes.					

The goal of the functional alternative belief is to open the possibility of other choices to the adolescent. Next, the adolescent and the clinician identify healthy alternative thoughts congruent with the new alternative belief.

111

Healthy Alternative Thoughts

Healthy alternative thoughts are meant to strengthen a particular functional alternative belief. To identify them, the clinician explores with the adolescent what type of thoughts he/she thinks would support the identified new belief. For example, you can ask the adolescent, "What thought(s) or words can you say to yourself to help you believe 'I can trust people sometimes?'" Let's say that the adolescent responds, "I will take a small step at a time with trust." This then becomes the healthy alternative thought for the identified functional alternative belief, as shown in the example below.

Functional Alternative Belief(s)	Healthy Alternative Thoughts	Functional Alternative Compensatory Strategy	Functional Reinforcing Behavior(s)	Specific Functional Treatment (Individual Treatment to Environment)	Validation, Clarification, Redirection (VCR)
I can trust people sometimes.	I will take a small step at a time with trust.				

You can see that the FTDF targets the new positive changes that the adolescent aspires to in a methodical manner—step-by-step. Thus, it is important to be thorough and to take your time when developing the FTDF. After determining the new alternative belief and accompanying thought, you and the adolescent then identify the functional alternative compensatory strategy that helps achieve and maintain this belief and thought.

Functional Alternative Compensatory Strategy

Functional alternative compensatory strategies encompass the MDT skills set that the adolescent employs to emotionally and behaviorally self-regulate, in order to balance his/her beliefs. This skills set includes mindfulness, acceptance, emotional defusion, cognitive defusion, and breathing exercises, as discussed in chapters 10 and 11. The clinician guides the adolescent in this section to incorporate mindfulness and other MDT strategies into the FTDF as shown in the example below.

Functional Alternative Belief(s)	Healthy Alternative Thoughts	Functional Alternative Compensatory Strategy	Functional Reinforcing Behavior(s)	Specific Functional Treatment (Individual Treatment to Environment)	Validation, Clarification, Redirection (VCR)
I can trust people sometimes.	I will take a small step at a time with trust.	Mindfulness, breathing, MDT skills set.			

After identifying the new belief, thought, and compensatory strategy, it is time to discuss behaviors that reinforce these new components in the adolescent's life.

Functional Reinforcing Behaviors

The functional reinforcing behavior replaces the previous dysfunctional behavior as a behavior that supports the new functional belief. You can refer to the COBB and the Client TFAB Collaborative Worksheet to review with the adolescent previous behaviors associated with the original endorsed belief(s). For example, on the completed COBB, the compound core belief "Everyone betrays my trust, I cannot trust anyone," identifies the corresponding behavior as "Threaten, punch." On the Client TFAB Collaborative Worksheet example, the adolescent translated and synthesized the belief and behavior into his/her own words as "If I don't trust you, I will threaten or punch you." When you are working at identifying alternative, healthy behaviors, you can ask the adolescent, "Now that you believe that you can trust people sometimes, how do you think you can act?" It is possible that the youth may say something like "I guess I can trust some people." Good. Consequently, at this time we would introduce the use of the Continuum of Trust (presented in chapter 12) to measure the adolescent's experiential trust and quantify success. The FTDF would look like this:

Functional Alternative Belief(s)	Healthy Alternative Thoughts	Functional Alternative Compensatory Strategy	Functional Reinforcing Behavior(s)	Specific Functional Treatment (Individual Treatment to Environment)	Validation, Clarification, Redirection (VCR)
I can trust people sometimes.	I will take a small step at a time with trust.	Mindfulness, breathing, MDT skills set.	Use trust scale situational.		

Because the change in behavior is incremental and unique to the adolescent, any trust shown would be interpreted as successful. It also demonstrates how the youth generalizes and transfers skills learned in individual sessions to external situations, which is the purpose of the next column of the FTDF.

Specific Functional Treatment: Individual Treatment to Environment

The specific functional treatment (individual treatment to environment) column illustrates how the skills learned and practiced in individual sessions with the clinician are self-initiated and implemented by the adolescent outside of the clinician's office. In the example that we have been illustrating ("I can trust people sometimes"), specific functional treatment skills learned in individual session that the youth could possibly incorporate in other situations could be mindfulness and the use of trust scales. In that case, the FTDF would look like this:

Functional Alternative Belief(s)	Healthy Alternative Thoughts	Functional Alternative Compensatory Strategy	Functional Reinforcing Behavior(s)	Specific Functional Treatment (Individual Treatment to Environment)	Validation, Clarification, Redirection (VCR)
I can trust people sometimes.	I will take a small step at a time with trust.	Mindfulness, breathing, MDT skills set.	Use trust scale situational.	Mindfulness, trust scales.	

The adolescent's application of MDT skills outside of the clinician's office requires the support of the youth's parent or caregiver, as discussed in chapter 12. Additionally, as has been mentioned throughout the book, acceptance and validation of the adolescent, and his/her grain of truth or perception of reality, are integral components of MDT that serve to redirect the youth toward healthier alternatives. We refer to this process as validation, clarification, and redirection (VCR).

Validation, Clarification, and Redirection

In MDT, the clinician *validates* the grain of truth in the adolescent's response, *clarifies* the content or meaning of the adolescent's response, and *redirects* the response by providing incrementally healthier alternatives. For example, to the compound core belief "Everyone betrays my trust, I cannot trust anyone," the clinician provides the adolescent validation with "You make sense not to trust people given your life experiences"; clarification follows with "It seems, though, that we have been honest with each other thus far in our relationship, so in this right here and now…"; and redirection completes the process with "Is it possible that you can, in this moment, trust me a little, say on a scale of 1 to 10?" The VCR process is discussed further in chapters 10 and 12. The VCR component completes the FTDF, as shown in the example below.

Functional Alternative Belief(s)	Healthy Alternative Thoughts	Functional Alternative Compensatory Strategy	Functional Reinforcing Behavior(s)	Specific Functional Treatment (Individual Treatment to Environment)	Validation, Clarification, Redirection (VCR)
I can trust people sometimes.	I will take a small step at a time with trust.	Mindfulness, breathing, MDT skills set.	Use trust scale situational.	Mindfulness, trust scales.	V: You make sense not to trust people given your life experiences. C: It seems, though, that we have been honest with each other thus far in our relationship, so in this right here and now… R: Is it possible that you can, in this moment, trust me a little, say on a scale of 1 to 10?

The FTDF contains more than one functional alternative belief, as you can see in the completed case conceptualization example in chapter 7. When completed, the FTDF becomes the clinician's blueprint for adolescent treatment, beginning with acknowledgment of the youth's grain of truth through the use of VCR. That means that when you implement the FTDF in treatment, you begin by applying the VCR (far right column) and proceed to the left to specific functional treatment (individual treatment to environment), and so on. From right to left, each column reinforces the next, gaining momentum and culminating with the functional alternative belief. The FTDF then becomes a cognitive and experiential process for the adolescent through which he/she can balance personal beliefs in order to construct a healthier belief system with functional corresponding behaviors.

Summary

In this chapter, we completed the last two steps of the case conceptualization: step VII, Mode Activation/Mode Deactivation; and step VIII, Functional Treatment Development Form. We encourage you to review your understanding of the mode activation and deactivation process by explaining it to colleagues. Go over the steps of validation, clarification, and redirection of the functional alternative belief. You can use a hypothetical situation to practice the process, and/or reexamine the examples presented in the book. Now that you have completed the case conceptualization, you have a comprehensive behavioral and emotional functional analysis of your adolescent and a treatment plan. Chapter 10 introduces you to the implementation of this plan.

Part III
MDT in Action

Chapter 10

MDT Treatment of Internalizing Disorders

After completing the MDT case conceptualization, you are ready to begin the MDT treatment process. This chapter introduces you to the MDT method of treating internalizing disorders, such as anxiety, depression, and trauma, in angry, aggressive, or oppositional adolescents.

Internalizing disorders are often so difficult for an adolescent to accept and manage that they can lead to feelings and beliefs that the adolescent experientially avoids. In other words, the adolescent goes out of his/her way to avoid experiencing hurtful feelings and beliefs. This avoidance can prompt the development of externalizing behaviors, such as aggression, parasuicide or other self-injurious behaviors, and also substance abuse, as a method of coping with and replacing the beliefs and/or feelings produced by the internalizing disorders. In other words, internalizing disorders can lead to externalizing disorders.

The MDT process can reduce the strength and frequency of the adolescent's internalizing disorders, as well as the externalizing aberrant behaviors. Following the MDT case conceptualization, the steps to implementing MDT as a psychotherapy treatment include the use of (1) mindfulness, (2) acceptance, (3) emotional defusion, (4) cognitive defusion, (5) validation, clarification, and redirection of the functional alternative beliefs, and (6) breathing mindfulness. We describe these components as follows:

- **Mindfulness** is to be fully in the moment. In other words, to see and accept things as they are, as we loosen our preoccupation with what we take to be the "self" and experience the richness of the present moment without judgment.

- **Acceptance** is to accept yourself as who, what, and where you are in the moment. This includes accepting pain, fears, and suffering as part of the human condition.

- **Emotional defusion** is to identify and experience emotional pain as occurring in a certain part of the body and to provide a complete description of the pain or numbness.

- **Cognitive defusion** is to allow thoughts that imprison and limit to occur without resistance, in order to move away from experiential avoidance of painful thoughts.

- **Validation, clarification, and redirection of functional alternative belief** (VCR of FAB) is to balance the adolescent's beliefs. This process derives from the Functional Treatment Development Form.

- **Breathing mindfulness** is used to center the adolescent and allow him or her to notice his or her breath and be in the moment.

Next, we will look at each of these MDT components through excerpts of sessions that illustrate their implementation in MDT treatment. But first, we want to point out that, although for discussion purposes, these elements are presented in a linear, sequential manner, the MDT process itself is synchronous and recursive. That is, we meet the adolescent where he or she is in the moment and implement the MDT component that best moves the process along at that particular time.

Mindfulness

As previously stated, mindfulness is to be fully in the moment, without judgment. We believe that in order to experience the richness of life and to begin the process of acceptance and defusion, the adolescent needs to be present to his/her current experience. However, some adolescents have difficulty truly being in the moment because many of them encounter some form of fear and anxiety as internalizing disorders. They become trapped in the T1 triggers (cognitive triggers or didactic learning) and T2 triggers (experiential triggers learned from life experiences). Mindfulness exercises help the adolescent become aware of himself/herself in the moment and reduce the strength of the anxiety, depression, or trauma. The exercises also assist in the acceptance of the self on a cognitive and an experiential/emotional level. This awareness and acceptance of self allow the adolescent to be more successful in MDT treatment. In chapter 11, we discuss the concept of MDT mindfulness further, and we provide a series of exercises to incorporate in sessions. However, basic breathing is a good place to start with an angry, aggressive, and oppositional adolescent, because breathing is a natural function of all human beings, and mindful breathing tends to relax, unclutter the brain, and reduce stress. For example,

Therapist: Let's take a second and do some breathing before we talk about anything.

Adolescent: Okay.

Therapist: Now, sit comfortably, feet on the floor, eyes closed if you want. Eyes open is okay, too. Inhale through your nose and exhale through your mouth. Just notice how your breath feels. Exhale and notice how it feels to exhale. Continue breathing at your own pace, inhale and exhale. Now, silently say "One" every time you exhale… inhale…silently say "One"… as you exhale.

[*Repeat this for five minutes.*]

Therapist: Open your eyes and allow yourself to get focused in this moment. Are you okay?

This simple exercise provides the opportunity for the adolescent to slow down physiologically, emotionally, and cognitively. The youth is then able to be more present in the session, which allows the clinician to introduce the concept of acceptance, described next.

Acceptance

Hayes (2004) identified psychological acceptance as one of the most important contextual change strategies. He defined acceptance as it refers to (1) the conscious abandonment of a direct change agenda in the key domains of private events, self, and history, and (2) an openness to experiencing thoughts and emotions as they are, not as the individual says they are expected to be. Dougher (1994) asserted that the key component of acceptance is letting go of one's control agenda and orienting the self toward valued actions. Acceptance, then, is not a goal in and of itself, but a method of empowering the individual to achieve life goals. Acceptance for the adolescent is also the ability to relate to and participate in difficult thoughts and emotions in the moment and to accept that life will contain these painful emotions and thoughts throughout one's lifetime. Here is an example of how to explore acceptance in an MDT session.

Adolescent: I feel like I am moving through these painful feelings and thoughts in a different way than I have in the past with other therapists. Now what?

Therapist: Well, let's talk about it. You have let yourself think these thoughts and feel the pain and you are still here. So, is it possible that you can accept that these painful thoughts and feelings are part of you, whether it sucks or not?

Adolescent: Yeah.

Therapist: And, it's clear you can experience them and not fall apart. Can you then commit yourself to move on with all of your pain and thoughts and not let them control your life?

Adolescent: I can try, but this isn't easy.

Therapist: You are right. It's not easy. However, you have just successfully accepted that they are part of you and you can move on with your life.

Adolescent: Yeah, I did.

Therapist: So, may there also be times when there are no painful feelings and thoughts?

Adolescent: Maybe, sometimes there are.

You can see how the clinician guides the adolescent through the process of acceptance of self, regardless of the experience of painful feelings, and most important the acceptance and acknowledgment that there are also times without those painful feelings. However, for many adolescents, the ability to experience other emotions besides painful feelings is difficult to attain or even imagine attaining. In MDT, we facilitate this process through emotional defusion.

Emotional Defusion

Emotional defusion addresses the specific underlying issues of pain or numbness of oppositional and traumatized adolescents who, as a result of years of abuse and neglect, cannot experience any feelings except pain. Many of these adolescents endorse beliefs such as "whenever I feel, it will be unpleasant." As a response to these painful emotions, these adolescents have separated themselves from their feelings, and they experience a lack of feeling or numbness in place of emotions. An essential part of emotional defusion is to guide the adolescent to identify in what part of the body he or she experiences the emotional pain by verbally guiding the adolescent to explore those feelings and their location in the body. For instance, the adolescent might say that the pain feels like a knot in "my stomach," that it feels like it's going to "explode." Even if the adolescent states that he/ she feels nothing or is numb, the clinician still guides the youth to address the exact area where the numbness exists in the body and then to identify the feelings associated with that numbness. The following is an illustration of how a therapist can employ emotional defusion in MDT therapy.

Therapist: In the last session, we discussed how you couldn't feel anything.

Adolescent: Yeah, I am numb. Empty.

Therapist: You endorsed the beliefs "Anything is better than feeling unpleasant" and "Whenever I hurt, I do what it takes to feel better." As "Always." Remember?

Adolescent: Yeah, so?

Therapist: Let's talk about your emptiness and numbness.

Adolescent: Okay.

Therapist: Tell me what your numbness feels like.

Adolescent: It feels like nothing.

Therapist: And, where is the nothing?

Adolescent: What do you mean, where?

Therapist: Where on or in your body do you notice the nothing—the emptiness and numbness?

Adolescent: [*Points to chest.*]

Therapist: Where on your chest?

Adolescent: Here, right in my chest.

Therapist: Describe how the numbness feels. What does the emptiness feel like in your chest?

Adolescent: It feels like an empty hole.

Therapist: What do you notice about this emptiness? Is it there to protect you from pain?

Adolescent: What pain?

Therapist: The pain of your past physical and emotional abuse. The pain you feel from your mother not being able to take care of you.

Adolescent: No, there was pain there but I cut it off.

Therapist: Okay, describe that pain that was there.

Adolescent: It was like a burning hole in my chest, like my heart had hot burning lava in there.

Therapist: Okay, let yourself experience that pain. The hot lava right here [*points to chest*]… right now. Let's sit with it.

By allowing the adolescent to experience these painful emotions in the moment, we are training him/her to not avoid them through dysfunctional behaviors or physiological reactions. Emotional pain in adolescents is often expressed as either intense physical pain or numbness in specific areas of their bodies. However, the youth's activated belief and corresponding core beliefs serve as experiential avoidance to the actual physical pain or numbness; that is, it becomes a conditioned response to avoid the actual feelings of pain. In MDT, we call the reversal of this process emotional defusion, because we attempt to defuse the link between the adolescent's emotional pain or numbness with the physiological pain in their body. The adolescents described in this book—angry, aggressive, and oppositional—are often still chronologically close to the experiences of trauma, emotional invalidation, or unavailability of parents or caregivers. As a result, the physical feelings can be more devastating than the cognitive ones. For these adolescents, emotional defusion is necessary in order for cognitive defusion to be possible and effective. The movement toward acceptance is also dependent upon the success of emotional defusion, because as long as the adolescent remains avoidant of personal pain or numbness, he/she cannot move into its acceptance. Through emotional defusion, the adolescent acquires more constructive ways of processing and managing pain. However, along with the emotions, there is a cognitive component that needs to be addressed in order for the adolescent to progress in MDT treatment. We target these intrusive cognitions through cognitive defusion.

Cognitive Defusion

The purpose of cognitive defusion is to help adolescents who are caught up in the content of their own cognitive activity to "defuse" from the literal meaning of those thoughts. Through cognitive defusion, the adolescent becomes more aware of thinking as an active, ongoing, relational process that is set both historically and situationally. The idea is to move the adolescent from the content of the verbal details of his/her life's story to the context of the adolescent in the moment. Cognitive defusion is based on a functional contextual theory of language and cognition called relational frame theory, or RFT (Hayes, Barnes-Holmes, & Roche, 2001). According to RFT, thoughts acquire their literal meaning and much of their focused emotive and behavior regulatory functions only because the social/verbal community establishes a context in which symbols relate mutually to other events and have functions based on these relations. Separating the adolescent from the content of painful thoughts in order to allow him/her to have a contextual experience of these thoughts reduces the power the contained words in the thoughts have over the adolescent. For example:

Therapist: What are the painful thoughts that go with this numbness and pain?

Adolescent: I am alone—no good. I am shit, like trash.

Therapist: Let yourself experience these thoughts and pain. You know that you have spent your life avoiding these painful thoughts and feelings. They are really hard as hell to deal with.

Adolescent: Yes, it really sucks sometimes that I have to live with pain and bad memories, but at least I can live with them and finally move on in my life.

The ability to defuse difficult and pain-inducing thoughts by separating the self from the cognition allows the adolescent to experience these distressing and painful thoughts in the moment, in order to process them effectively. This activity also sets the stage for validation, clarification, and redirection of the functional alternative belief.

Balancing Beliefs

Validation, clarification, and redirection (VCR) of the functional alternative belief (FAB) is what separates MDT from all other CBT or third wave methodologies. Validation involves looking for the grain of truth in the adolescent's perceptions or beliefs. Clarification is the process of clarifying the content of the adolescent's response and requires the clinician to verbally guide the adolescent by validating each response and moving toward a redirection. Thus, the clinician verbally moves the adolescent to the possibility of accepting the functional alternative belief in the moment. In other words, the idea is to verbally reinforce or validate each statement throughout the session until the clinician can reach a point of agreement for redirection toward the functional alternative belief. That is, the clinician's goal for redirection is for the adolescent to realize that his/her functional alternative belief could be true to some degree in the moment.

The clinician can measure the adolescent's possible acceptance of the new belief on a scale of 1 to 10 by verbally asking the youth or using one of the continuum scales presented in chapter 12. If, for instance, the adolescent agrees that he/she could be okay while experiencing unpleasant feelings in the moment, you ask how much could he/she deal with unpleasant feelings and be okay on a scale of 1 to 10.

Therapist: It's not easy, but you have just successfully accepted that they [painful feelings] are part of you and you can move on with your life.

Adolescent: Yes, I did.

Therapist: So, you agree that you can experience painful or numb feelings and be okay at times?

Adolescent: This time.

Therapist: It makes sense that you are in therapy given your history. Your childhood was filled with hurt and anger and being on your own most of the time.

Adolescent: You know it.

Therapist: So you being here with all these feelings of anger and hurt makes sense and it is where you need to be, but you also can experience your painful thoughts and emotions and be okay.

Adolescent: I don't know if I can.

Therapist: I mean right now in this moment, you can experience unpleasant feelings and be okay.

Adolescent: Right now, yeah.

Therapist: Tell me how much you really believe you are okay experiencing these painful thoughts and feelings on a scale of 1 to 10, right now.

Adolescent: Maybe a 6.

Therapist: Are you sure a 6?

Adolescent: Yeah.

Therapist: So, 60 percent of the time, you, in this moment, are able to experience unpleasant feelings and be okay.

Adolescent: Yeah, I need more work with this shit, though.

Therapist: You will keep working on it, because it works and you are important and can experience some good stuff in life.

Adolescent: Okay.

Therapist: Can I ask one more thing? You had endorsed the belief "Always," for "Whenever I hurt, I do what it takes to feel better." Right?

Adolescent: Yeah.

Therapist: So, before, what did you do to feel better?

Adolescent: Fight, drink, smoke weed. You know, stuff like that.

Therapist: Okay, but you just experienced painful thoughts, hurtful feelings and that hot lava—and you said you could deal with it 60 percent of the time, right here and now. Right?

Adolescent: Yeah, so?

Therapist: So, is it possible to hurt and be okay with it in this moment?

Adolescent: Yeah, right now I can.

Therapist: So right here and right now in this moment, you can hurt and be okay and not have to fight, drink, smoke weed or any other stuff?

Adolescent: Yeah, right now with you.

Therapist: That's where it starts. Good work for today! We'll continue working on this next session so you can feel numbness and pain and be okay in the moment.

The fact that the adolescent experienced unpleasant feelings in the session and was able to accept and defuse them is the stepping-stone for the youth to agree to some degree that he/she can do it again in the future. This process targets both the cognitive and the experiential learning of the adolescent within the MDT session. The intense emotional work accomplished in an MDT session can be stabilized with a breathing mindfulness exercise, as shown next.

Breathing Mindfulness

It is important to help the adolescent remain centered after an MDT session. Therefore, a breathing mindfulness exercise is recommended at the conclusion of the session.

> *Therapist:* Okay, let's end the session with a breathing mindfulness exercise. Close your eyes and notice your breath—the part of your breath after you inhale, right before you exhale. You actually stop breathing for that nanosecond in between inhale and exhale. Just inhale and notice the peace of that brief nanosecond prior to exhaling...exhale. Let's just do this for 10 breaths.

[The adolescent takes 10 slow breaths]

> *Therapist:* How do you feel now?
>
> *Adolescent:* Really okay.
>
> *Therapist:* Try practicing that every day for 10 breaths and let me know how it works out.
>
> *Adolescent:* Okay.
>
> *Therapist:* Great work. See you next week.

Ending a session with breathing mindfulness leaves the adolescent centered and less anxious and/or upset about facing feared painful emotions. In our experience, adolescents have referred to the end-of-session breathing exercises as "perfect" and "peaceful," especially after a difficult session. However, a breathing exercise can also be used at the beginning of the session to set the tone or at any time during the session, as needed.

One More Time

It is important to understand the validation, clarification, and redirection (VCR) methodology and its effectiveness both in and out of session. Remember that the adolescent's functional alternative belief (FAB) must be validated in the moment, whether he/she is in session or out of session and in the "real world." The out-of-session application is clearly delineated in the specific functional treatment (individual treatment to environment) column of the Functional Treatment Development Form (FTDF), which recommends how MDT is to be generalized in the adolescent's home, school, or living environment by parents, teachers, or caregivers. This specific step is designed to assure generalization of the T1 and T2 triggers outside of the therapy session environment. Let's review what these concepts look like in a session with an adolescent who endorsed the belief "Anything is better than feeling unpleasant" with "Always." Notice how the adolescent's belief is converted by the therapist and the adolescent as the following FAB: "I can feel unpleasant at times and be okay with life."

Therapist:	It is clear that you have been through a lot of bad times in your life that have caused you pain. It makes sense that when you have let yourself feel, it has been a painful process for you.
Adolescent:	Yes, so?
Therapist:	So tell me, when you allow yourself to experience painful thoughts and feelings, what feelings or sensations do you notice?
Adolescent:	I hurt all over. My head buzzes and feels like it's gonna explode. My chest feels empty and numb.
Therapist:	Okay. Just sit and let yourself feel your hurting head and your numb chest. What thoughts go with the pain?
Adolescent:	I am alone and no one gives a fuck about me.
Therapist:	That is a lot to carry for you. It would be a lot for anyone to carry.
Adolescent:	It fucking hurts.
Therapist:	As you allow yourself to experience these painful thoughts and emotions, do you notice that you are dealing with them and you are still here and okay? They hurt, but you are okay.
Adolescent:	Yeah, I'm still here for now; even though the feelings hurt.
Therapist:	Okay, right here in this moment. Can you accept that you have these painful thoughts and emotions at times, but you can still move on with your life?
Adolescent:	Sometimes, maybe I can.
Therapist:	On a scale of 1 to 10, how much do you believe that you can accept yourself in the moment and move forward with your life?
Adolescent:	Five, I think.
Therapist:	Okay, right here in this moment, you can feel hurt and 50 percent of the time be okay and move on?
Adolescent:	Yes.
Therapist:	Good, you have begun to not avoid your feelings or your thoughts and still get on with your life.

The above example illustrates an alternative to change in the adolescent's conscious and out-of-awareness learning through MDT. Again, the out-of-session work is imperative to assure the long-term success of MDT treatment. This also requires familiarizing the adolescent's parents or caregivers with relevant aspects of MDT methodology to ensure a successful transition for the youth. Therefore (as further discussed in chapter 12), whether working with an outpatient or a residential inpatient, the MDT clinician needs to accept that his/her work with the adolescent extends beyond the office to the family or caregiver.

Your Turn

Now, let's see how you are internalizing the MDT methodology. The example below integrates mindfulness, emotional defusion, cognitive defusion, acceptance, and balancing beliefs with validation, clarification, and redirection of the functional alternative belief. Please identify which particular MDT skills are being practiced throughout the example below:

Therapist: It seems that you had a rough weekend, according to your mother.

Adolescent: She exaggerates sometimes.

Therapist: Did she this time?

Adolescent: Well, I did cut myself and smoke some weed.

Therapist: You know, I think we should focus on you now in this moment, so can we do some mindfulness breathing?

Adolescent: I am not into it right now. It won't work.

Therapist: Since you are breathing anyway, why not breathe together?

Adolescent: Okay, okay.

Therapist: Inhale through your mouth and exhale through your nose. Notice the brief nano-second that you are not breathing. Let yourself experience that brief moment of peace and as you exhale, silently say, "One." Good. Inhale. Experience a moment of peace. Exhale to "One."

[The breathing was repeated for about 4 minutes]

Therapist: Okay, now what do you notice that you are feeling emotionally?

Adolescent: Nothing—I am empty and numb.

Therapist: Can you tell me where your emptiness is in your body?

Adolescent: [*Points to her chest, her heart.*]

Therapist: Describe the feeling of emptiness and numbness in your chest and heart.

Adolescent: It is like it is cold and I am feeling nothing there.

Therapist: As you look deeper in your heart and chest, what might you feel behind your emptiness?

Adolescent: You mean the pain and deep ache like my heart is going to blow up?

Therapist: Yes, that's it. Can you let yourself go behind the numbness and feel that pain right here?

[*Adolescent begins to weep and appears to be experiencing painful emotions.*]

Therapist: Can you tell me some of the painful thoughts that are attached to these painful feelings?

Adolescent: I am shit, nothing, worthless. Life is a waste and no one gives a fuck about me.

Therapist: Good, but what do all these words really mean? They are just words.

Adolescent: Maybe so, but they hurt.

Therapist: Look at the word "worthless." Let's repeat it together 10 times. "Worthless, worthless, worthless…"

[*Adolescent repeats "worthless" 10 times with therapist.*]

Therapist: It sounds silly, but it *is* silly in a way, because it is only a word. Nothing but a word. You have all these emotions attached to this word.

Adolescent: Okay, so?

Therapist: So, you were able to sit and experience your painful emotions and your painful thoughts and you are still here and okay, right?

Adolescent: Yes, but I am feeling anxious.

Therapist: Okay. You now have experienced these painful thoughts and feelings and are only a little anxious. Right?

Adolescent: Yes.

Therapist: You can decide that if you experience these painful feelings or thoughts you can survive. But then, these feelings might come and go throughout your life. Can you accept that might be true?

Adolescent: I don't like it, but I can accept it.

Therapist: So, are you ready to move forward with your life together with your painful feelings and emotions, right now?

Adolescent: It isn't easy, but I will try.

Therapist: Is that a yes?

Adolescent: Yes.

Therapist: Good. What belief is activating and setting off these painful thoughts and emotions?

Adolescent: I can't deal with unpleasant feelings, and anything is better than feeling unpleasant or feeling pain.

Therapist: You endorsed those beliefs with a "4" or "Always," correct?

Adolescent: Yes.

Therapist: You realize that right here today, you were able to deal with your painful thoughts and emotions and were okay?

Adolescent: Yes, but I still feel my heart pounding.

Therapist: That's okay. But you now know that there are times, like right here and right now, that you can deal with your pain. So, on a scale of 1 to 10, how much do you think that it is possible for you to deal with your painful beliefs?

Adolescent: Around a 5 or so.

Therapist: Great. So 50 percent of the time, you can experience these painful feelings and thoughts and be okay with them.

Adolescent: Yes, I think I can.

Therapist: That is amazing! You have found a possible alternative, 50 percent of the time, to cutting or smoking weed.

Adolescent: That's what I said.

Therapist: Great work. Can we finish our session today with a breathing exercise?

Adolescent: Yes, I want to do that.

[The same breathing mindfulness exercise from the beginning of the session is repeated for five minutes to alleviate her anxiety and complete the session.]

Therapist: You feeling okay now?

Adolescent: Yes, better.

Therapist: On a scale of 1 to 10, where is your anxiety?

Adolescent: Only a 1.5.

Therapist: Okay, great work!

This session addressed the behavioral function of this adolescent female's cutting and drug usage—the pain and numbness that hide and protect her deeper emotional pain. She experienced functional alternative behaviors to address her pain, as well as mindfulness, emotional defusion, cognitive defusion, and VCR of the FAB. You can check the accuracy of your responses by reviewing the completed worksheet provided in Appendix B of this book.

Summary

MDT helps the adolescent understand how to interrupt the moods, emotions, and anger that imprison and interfere with life and treatment. The MDT treatment process is not linear but synchronous, which means that working with an adolescent in therapy is like a dance. And, as in a dance, practice makes you better but you might need to adjust during a performance. For example, depending on the moment, you might have to employ the acceptance component following the cognitive and emotional defusion, or vice versa. Remember, it is a dance and you need to be there in the moment to be successful as an MDT clinician. The next chapter presents a series of mindfulness exercises used in MDT treatment.

Chapter 11

MDT Mindfulness Exercises

Now that you have an understanding of many of the MDT components, we want to take a moment to explore the use of mindfulness in MDT. In therapeutic treatment, mindfulness is the context in which the other elements of MDT (acceptance; emotional defusion; cognitive defusion; validation, clarification, and redirection of the functional alternative belief; and breathing mindfulness) occur. In fact, mindfulness is incorporated into all aspects of MDT—whether it is therapy or the administration of a Fear Assessment or CCBQ-S.

You may already have a mindfulness practice in your life. Or perhaps you are new to this mindset and are wondering why it is such a vital part of MDT. In this chapter, we illustrate the integration of mindfulness in MDT treatment and provide a variety of exercises you can readily incorporate in therapy, and in your own life. However, we do not attempt to provide an exhaustive discussion of mindfulness in this book, nor do we present ourselves as experts on the subject of mindfulness itself. We simply offer examples of how to integrate mindfulness, in the moment, into MDT in the treatment of angry, aggressive, and oppositional adolescents. We encourage the reader to refer to the wealth of information currently available on mindfulness. We believe mindfulness is an experiential process; therefore, the overall purpose of this chapter is to provide a series of mindfulness exercises for you to practice and ultimately use in MDT sessions. The exercises themselves contain many specific MDT skills, such as emotional and cognitive defusion. Consequently, they also help the adolescent develop MDT skills in an experientially mindful manner.

Why Mindfulness in MDT?

As previously noted, mindfulness is to be fully present in the moment. In other words, to see and accept things as they are, as we let go of our fixation on what we take to be the "self" and experience the richness of the here and now, objectively. Mindfulness is an essential component of MDT for several reasons. It helps train the adolescent to be fully aware of his/her self in the moment; this awareness begins to reduce the fear and avoidance of MDT. It also helps the adolescent become more open to the process of emotional defusion, cognitive defusion, and acceptance. Mindfulness reduces stress and anxiety, which, in essence, reduces resistance-based avoidance in the adolescent.

In MDT, resistance or opposition represents the adolescent's internal struggle: attempting to avoid contact with his or her painful thoughts and emotions. In other words, resistance is the internal behavioral manifestation of opposition expressed through avoidance, and it should be expected when working with the type of adolescent population MDT treats. If you think of resistance as a naturally occurring behavior implemented by the adolescent for protection from actual physical and emotional pain, then you can perceive resistance as a function of experiential avoidance. In MDT, this becomes a teaching event for the clinician and a learning opportunity for the adolescent. Most adolescents exhibit some form of resistance or opposition to the change process of MDT—this is simply a form of self-protection against the pain or numbness that the youth desires to avoid at all costs. Remember that the adolescent's externalizing disorders were developed in order to cope with hurtful beliefs and feelings that are the hallmarks of internalizing disorders. Therefore, mindfulness is an essential component of MDT because it helps reduce or eliminate the adolescent's resistance to and avoidance of painful experiences and sometimes even life in general.

However, the implementation of mindfulness with adolescents, particularly angry, aggressive, or oppositional adolescents, can be a challenge. Many adolescents may not want to participate in an activity possibly perceived as "corny" or "silly." Others may feel uncomfortable or too vulnerable closing their eyes around anyone, much less a clinician. Well, who can blame them? The path to lowering these perceptions of vulnerability and distrust rests with the clinician, as presented in the next section.

Mindfulness and the Clinician

We believe mindfulness is a state of being for both the clinician and the youth; therefore you need to practice mindfulness yourself in order to teach the practice to your adolescent client. This is not a new concept, as mindfulness is also encouraged by mindfulness-based cognitive therapy (MBCT), dialectical behavior therapy (DBT), functional analytic psychotherapy (FAP), and acceptance and commitment therapy (ACT). In fact, Hayes (2004) poignantly synthesized the idea of a clinician and client's dual mindfulness immersion as "swimming in the same stream." Again, the clinician needs to experience the benefits of mindfulness firsthand in order to approach the adolescent from an honest position. This facilitates teaching the adolescent how this practice can assist in effective management of thinking and emotions, and consequently provide cognitive and emotional balance in his/her life. The clinician's personal mindfulness experience also allows for a greater understanding of where the adolescent is "coming from," because in MDT the clinician needs to figuratively climb into the adolescent's thinking and beliefs and make mindfulness real and important. This is simply a means of joining and fully understanding the grain of truth in the adolescent's thinking, beliefs, and behaviors. According to the theory of modes (Beck, 1996), the adolescent's perceptions constitute his/her context of reality. Hence, the clinician must fully understand these perceptions as manifested in the adolescent's thinking and beliefs. In this chapter, we present a series of mindfulness exercises—from basic breathing and relaxation to imagery, balancing, and acceptance exercises. We recommend that you practice each exercise yourself before guiding the adolescent to participate. When you are comfortable practicing mindfulness, you are ready to guide adolescents in its practice.

Using Mindfulness Exercises

The breathing and imagery exercises in this chapter are examples of the type of exercises we integrate in MDT that we have found effective in the treatment of angry, aggressive, and oppositional adolescents. We recommend that you introduce each exercise carefully, based on the therapeutic readiness of the adolescent, in order to not create more fear or anxiety for the youth by going too quickly or skipping steps. Make sure that you are familiar with the adolescent's beliefs and fears. For example, if the youth is fearful of the ocean, you would not introduce exercise 5 (Ocean Imagery) at the onset of treatment. Take a moment to process the experience with the adolescent after each exercise before continuing with the session. You can use mindfulness exercises at the beginning, middle, or conclusion of any MDT session. There may also be times when you choose to implement a full session on mindfulness to simply reduce anxiety, depression, and/or anger. The practice and processing of mindfulness in MDT sessions empowers the adolescent to self-implement the skills out of session.

The exercises in the next pages are provided as they are presented directly to the youth. However, as previously indicated, we want you to practice each one first (on your own) before you integrate it into an MDT session. For best results, read each exercise in its entirety, before practicing it yourself. Once you have practiced it, notice how you feel emotionally and cognitively. Are you more relaxed? Can you think more clearly? Do you have more energy? Again, it is critical that you be familiar and comfortable with the process before you ask the adolescent to participate. A good way to start is with a relaxation and breathing exercise, such as the one below, to help quiet the mind. This exercise is also good for fostering self-esteem.

Exercise 1: Relaxation Is a State of Mindfulness

When you are presenting this exercise to an adolescent, you can make it relevant by adding references to experiences congruent to the youth.

- *You know your mind is chattering when you are in school, talking to your family, or even playing sports with your friends. Your mind, like all parts of your body, needs to rest, right? Did you ever notice how sometimes your mind or the chatter tells you that you can't do something? Like pass a test, stop drinking, or stop fighting? You know, the negative and busy chatter we all have in our minds. Here's an exercise to help you relax and quiet your mind. First, sit in a comfortable chair and let your hands rest on your lap. Just notice your breathing. Then silently repeat the following: "I am better than good..." You might feel silly or think this is corny, but try it and see for yourself. "I am better than good..." Then one word, "I." If other thoughts come into your head, it is okay. Just focus on "I" yet do not struggle...allow other thoughts to come and go and return to "I." Now go to "Am." For 10 breaths think only of "Am." Shift from "Am" to the space between "I" and "Am"...the nothingness in between. Let yourself just remain in the blank and empty space in between these words. After 10 breaths switch back to "Am" for 5 breaths...then shift to "Better." Just stay with "Better" in your mind's eye for 10 breaths...now back to the space between "Am" and "Better." Stay in the nothingness of this space...Breathe...10 full breaths. And back to "Better"...5 full breaths...shift to the word... "Than." Each exhale silently say "Than." 10 full breaths...then again shift to the space between "Better" and "Than"...try to empty all other thoughts and float in that empty space for 10 breaths...Now back to "Than" for 5 breaths...every exhale..."Thhhhhhaaaaaaaaaaaaannnnn." Now shift to "Good." Every exhale silently say "Gooooooood"...10 full breaths...nice. Now shift to the space between "Than" and "Good" ...stay in that emptiness for 10 breaths...inhale...exhale...Now back to "Goooooooooood" for 5 full breaths...You may slowly bring yourself back to the moment or continue with the breathing until you are ready.*

Process the experience with the adolescent after the exercise. Ask what it was like for him/her during the exercise. Notice the youth's level of comfort, stress, and disclosure. Valuable information is obtained about the adolescent through his/her interpretation of the experience, however brief the discussion may be. The after-exercise processing also provides guidance for the clinician regarding the therapeutic choice of future mindfulness exercises to incorporate in sessions.

Chapter 10 presented how MDT teaches the adolescent to balance beliefs through the validation, clarification, and redirection of the functional alternative belief. This process is enhanced by also teaching the adolescent to balance his/her whole being, as in the next exercise.

Exercise 2: Balance Yourself

Explain to the adolescent that MDT teaches you how to balance beliefs, but first you need to balance and center your thoughts, feelings, and body. Here is an exercise to help achieve this balance of self:

- *Locate your thinking: find where exactly your thoughts are generated in your mind.*

- *Notice your feelings—find where they are centered in your body.*

- *Picture a circle surrounding your thoughts.*

- *Picture another circle surrounding your feelings.*

- *Just take a moment to notice these two circles within yourself.*

- *Slowly allow each circle to merge with the other until there is no distance between them.*

- *Slowly merge them until they are one circle.*

- *Hold that for a few seconds and...inhale...then exhale.*

After balancing himself/herself through this exercise, it is easier for the adolescent to balance his/her compound core beliefs. To help the youth (and you) become more comfortable with breathing and relaxation as well as with the process of letting go, the next exercise combines breathing with progressive muscle relaxation.

Exercise 3: Conscious Breathing

Tell the adolescent that this experience is an exercise in conscious breathing and progressive muscle relaxation that helps you learn to relax by "going inside and letting go of all outside distractions."

- *Please sit comfortably in your chair with your back straight. Place both feet flat on the floor, with your legs uncrossed, arms resting along the sides of your body with your hands in your lap, palms up. Now gently close your eyes. Begin to relax your body and focus on your breathing. As you begin to focus your attention on your breathing, your awareness of external surroundings will decrease. In fact, any distractions that you may hear will only help you to relax even more deeply. By breathing deeply you are now becoming aware of internal sensations. And as you relax even more your pulse slows, your breathing slows, you begin to withdraw from the outside world, and you can direct your attention to any suggestions you are given. (PAUSE.)*

- *Notice how easily your breath flows in and flows out as it settles into its own natural rhythm. Feel how relaxed you are becoming as you simply allow the breath to flow in and out. You are becoming even more relaxed with each breath, breathing effortlessly. Another breath in and out. All tension is being released now; all tension is just melting away. Your body is becoming more and more relaxed as you continue to follow the breath in and out. You feel so safe and secure as you rest here in pure and simple relaxation. (PAUSE.)*

- *Now allow yourself to imagine a warm light, the brightest sunlight from the most beautiful and peaceful place you can imagine. You are drawn to this sunlight and the sunlight is drawn to you. Allow this warm and soothing sunlight to surround you; it is not hot or threatening, only calm and steady. The sunlight will fill you with relaxation. Now slowly merge with the sunlight…*

- *Slowly and effortlessly you and the sunlight become one.*

- *It's true that you always breathe without needing to even think about it. Most of the time you aren't even aware of your breathing; it just happens all by itself. The lungs take air in and then automatically, the lungs release the air. During breathing, the oxygen you take in replaces carbon dioxide in just the right amount to nourish and cleanse your blood and all the cells of your body. Concentrate on your breathing now. Allow your chest to expand fully and completely. Begin to breathe slowly and deeply, with the chest relaxed. As the air moves into the lungs, the belly will expand a bit until it is comfortably full. Now relax and let the breath go by exhaling. And as you exhale, feel the release of tension, feel the relaxation, feel the effortless movement of air out of your lungs. This is the natural way to breathe. Let your body breathe all by itself, slowly and naturally. Let your breathing take on its own natural rhythm, its own pace, without controlling it, without forcing it. I'll be quiet as you allow your body to breathe on its own for a few moments. (PAUSE.)*

- *You're now going to use your breath to relax even more. Breathe in deeply and as you slowly exhale, mentally direct the breath into your head and facial area. Feel the breath fill your head and face, filling it with pure relaxation. Your scalp relaxes, your eyes relax, all your facial muscles relax; your jaw relaxes and your mouth opens a bit and relaxes. Another breath in and as you slowly exhale, now direct the breath into your neck and shoulder area. Feel the breath fill your neck and shoulders, filling them with pure relaxation. Your neck and shoulders are completely relaxed. Another breath in, and as you slowly exhale, now direct the breath into your chest and back. Feel the breath fill your chest and back, filling them with pure relaxation. Your chest and back are completely relaxed. Another breath in…*

- *As you slowly exhale, now direct the breath into your arms, wrists, and fingers. Feel the breath fill your arms, wrists, and fingers, filling them with pure relaxation. Your arms, wrists, and fingers are completely relaxed. Another breath in, and as you slowly exhale, now direct the breath into your stomach. Feel the breath fill your stomach, filling it with pure relaxation. Your stomach is completely relaxed. Another breath in, and as you slowly exhale, now direct the breath into your upper legs. Feel your breath now fill your upper legs, filling them with pure relaxation. Your upper legs are now completely relaxed. Another breath in, and as you slowly exhale, now direct the breath into your knees, legs, and ankles. Feel the breath fill your knees, legs, and ankles, filling them with pure relaxation. Your knees, legs, and ankles are completely relaxed. Another breath in, and as you slowly exhale, now direct the breath into your feet and toes. Feel the breath fill your feet and toes, filling them with pure relaxation. Your feet and toes are completely relaxed. Take a moment to notice the sense of peace and relaxation that now fills your whole body—that fills every cell within you. You feel so calm, so peaceful. Drift and float into a deeper and deeper level of total relaxation as I count from five to one...5...4...3...going deeper...2...1...deeper still. You feel as though a heavy weight has been lifted off your shoulders. This is the deepest state of relaxation you have ever experienced. (PAUSE.)*

- *You can return to this state of pure and simple relaxation any time you want to calm any feelings of hostility, any feelings of anxiety, any feelings of agitation, or any feelings of sadness, just by focusing on the breath and relaxing each part of your body one at a time just as you did here. (PAUSE.)*

- *Bring your attention back to your breath. Take a slow, deep breath in and gently release. Another breath in and release. Begin to become aware of your body resting comfortably in your chair. Become more in touch with your body as you begin to move your fingers and toes.*

- *Become aware of your surroundings as you take another breath in and release. You are now ready to return to full waking consciousness; as I count from five to one you will feel refreshed, you will feel alert, and you will open your eyes when I say the number one...5...4...feeling refreshed...3...2...feeling alert...and 1. Open your eyes.*

As you and the adolescent develop the ability for conscious breathing, there will come a moment when breath itself becomes subtle, becomes smooth, and produces happiness and joy. From that time onward, indulging in thoughts while practicing conscious breathing is a kind of suffering. That is, you (and hopefully the adolescent) will "elect" to be with the breath and attain an intense mindfulness in each moment of breath. What this means in MDT is that through simply practicing conscious breathing, you can obtain inner quiet and a still, mindful mind.

In order to facilitate the process of acceptance in MDT, the next exercise helps the adolescent use acceptance as a mindfulness technique—in other words, be in the moment and accept himself/herself as who he/she is in the moment. This skill is later transferred to other areas in MDT treatment.

Exercise 4: The Fog and the Valley

- *Please sit comfortably in your chair with your back straight. Place both feet flat on the floor, with your legs uncrossed, arms resting along the sides of your body with hands in your lap, palms up. You may keep your eyes open or close them. However you feel comfortable.*

- *You are sitting in a warm, sunny valley. You notice how the sun warms your body and the light shines through the trees and glistens on the surrounding mountains. You feel the peace, the quiet, and the warmth of the sun. As you inhale and exhale, peace flows through you. Now you notice some fog beginning to show over the tops of the mountains. You remain calm, holding the warmth of the sun and the peace of the valley.*

- *The fog now moves over the mountain and begins to fill the trees. Now, as you see the fog, you know you will be engulfed as well, in the cool, misty fog. You now accept that the fog will cover you and you can accept it as it is. You accept the fog as it covers you. You feel the coolness and the dampness, but you are warmed by letting yourself experience the fog and accepting that just as it rolled in, it will go away. Stay where you are with your peace with the fog. Inhale. Exhale.*

- *As you accept the fog and yourself as you are, the fog begins to roll out and you begin to see the sun as it shines over the mountain tops. Breathe. The sunlight now glistens on the trees. The fog is gone and you now accept the warmth of the sun. Inhale. Exhale.*

- *Experience the warmth of acceptance and peace. Now, stay with the sun, and with acceptance, and at your own pace begin to wake up. Slowly let yourself come back and keep the peace within you.*

Remember to process the experience with the adolescent. You may notice that the trust in the therapeutic alliance increases as the youth becomes more comfortable with himself/herself and you. This, in turn, can decrease the level of guardedness the adolescent may have toward treatment. Fostering a sense of relaxation and inner peace, as in the next exercise, facilitates the process of MDT for the adolescent.

Exercise 5: Ocean Imagery

- *Please sit comfortably in your chair with your back straight. Place both feet flat on the floor, with your legs uncrossed, arms resting along the sides of your body with hands in your lap, palms up. Now gently close your eyes. Begin to relax your body and focus on your breathing. As you begin to focus your attention on your breathing, your awareness of external surroundings will decrease. In fact, any distractions that you might hear will only help you to relax even more deeply. By breathing deeply you are now becoming aware of internal sensations. And as you relax even more, your pulse slows, your breathing slows, you begin to withdraw from the outside world, and you can direct your attention to any suggestions you are given. (PAUSE.)*

- *Notice how easily your breath flows in and flows out, as it settles into its own natural rhythm. Feel how relaxed you are becoming as you simply allow the breath to flow in and out. You are becoming even more relaxed with each breath, breathing so effortlessly. Another breath in and out. All tension is being released now, all tension is just melting away. Your body is becoming more and more relaxed as you continue to follow the breath in and out. You feel so safe and secure as you rest here in pure and simple relaxation. (PAUSE.)*

- *Now allow yourself to imagine a warm light, the brightest sunlight, from the most beautiful and peaceful place you can imagine. You are drawn to this sunlight and the sunlight is drawn to you. Allow this warm and soothing sunlight to surround you; it is not hot or threatening, only calm and steady. The sunlight will fill you with relaxation. Now slowly merge with the sunlight…*

- *Feel your heart beating in perfect rhythm with the light; for it is this energy that gives you life that beats within your heart. (PAUSE.)*

- *Allow yourself to now imagine that you are standing at the ocean shore on a bright and sunny summer morning. Notice how clear this scene becomes when you add all the details and how good it feels to be here. Sense how warm the sand is beneath your feet—just the perfect temperature. Allow your toes to sink in a bit. You may safely lie down on the sand or take a walk by the surf. Listen now to the sound of the waves moving onto the shore and moving out again; watch them roll in and out; gently and easily they ebb and flow. Above you, now you can also hear the sound of a seagull's cry as it glides though the air. Watch it as it flies out of sight over the horizon. As your gaze follows the seagull, you notice several dolphins swimming in the distance. See them jumping in and out of the waves as they move through the ocean. Notice the scent of the ocean air. Take a deep breath as you inhale the ocean scent—so fresh and clean. Feel the ocean breeze on your skin now; it is slightly cool, but the sun is warm and soothing. A few clouds drift across the sky; a sky that goes on forever and the bright sunlight that reaches you shining down between the clouds allows you to feel so warm and relaxed, so peaceful. (PAUSE.)*

- *Allow this warm and soothing sunlight to flow through you, relaxing every muscle, every tissue, and every cell in your body. As it flows through you from head to toe, allow it to completely relax each part of your body. As the light begins to flow through the scalp and forehead, feel all stress simply fade away. The light continues to flow through the eyes and the eyes become relaxed and heavier. The sunlight now flows down over the temples and face, relaxing the lips and jaw and continues to flow through the front of the neck. At the same time it flows down the back of your head, neck and shoulders. Allow gravity to pull your shoulders into their natural position. (PAUSE.)*

- *The mind may wander and drift or it may become a bit drowsy or foggy. Whatever happens is completely perfect. You will still hear the sound of my voice as it becomes a comfortable sound in the background. My words will soon blend into one another and flow into your mind easily, so you will be free from having to listen to the words, as the subconscious understands their meaning anyway. And the mind simply relaxes, letting go of all thoughts, all concerns, as you allow yourself to simply relax in the moment. All fear, guilt, and self-blame are now released in this moment. Allow all problems, pressures, and stresses that have built up to simply melt away, just melt away. Drift and float into a deeper and deeper level of total relaxation as I count from five to one...5...4...3...going deeper...2...1...deeper still. (PAUSE.)*

- *Allow the sunlight to continue to flow through the elbows, through the wrists, and out through the fingers. Your breathing becomes deeper now. With each more relaxing breath, feel your back resting more firmly against your chair. As the light flows down the back, all the muscles and tendons relax and your back settles into its natural position. The sunlight continues to flow through the waist, stomach, upper legs, now moving through the thighs, knees, legs and into the ankles. As the light moves out through the toes, it releases all stress, all concerns, all worries that have caused you tension by being locked up in the body. Now feel all the accumulated stress and tension totally released from your body with each new breath you take—breathing slowly and gently, inhaling and exhaling. With each beat of your heart, feel yourself going deeper into relaxation, completely free of all tension, all worries, all concerns. Remain in the deep relaxation for a few moments, staying with the beating of your heart and relaxing even more deeply as you follow the gentle rhythm of its slow and steady beating, while I am silent for a few moments. (PAUSE.)*

- *You can return to this state of pure and simple relaxation any time you want to calm any feelings of hostility, any feelings of anxiety, any feelings of agitation, or any feelings of sadness. (PAUSE.)*

- *Bring your attention back to the ocean shore you have been standing or lying upon and to the warm and soothing sunlight that has been flowing through your body. Allow this image to slowly fade away, slowly fade away as you now bring your attention back to your breath. Take a slow, deep breath in and gently release. Another breath in and release. Begin to become aware of your body resting comfortably in your chair. Become more in touch with your body as you begin to move your fingers and toes. Become aware of your surroundings as you breathe in and release. You are now ready to return to full waking consciousness, as I count from five to one. You will feel refreshed, you will feel alert, and you will open your eyes when I say the number one...5...4...feeling refreshed...3....2...feeling alert...and 1. Open your eyes.*

Mindfulness exercises are infused into MDT treatment to reduce the adolescent's anxiety, anger, and feelings of being unsettled. Through practice, they become portable tools that the individual can access throughout his/her life.

Adapting the Mindfulness Exercises

The exercises presented in this chapter constitute only a small sampling of the many available for MDT mindfulness. As the MDT process unfolds, you can incorporate other components as dictated by the therapeutic needs of the adolescent. For example, you can help the adolescent internalize his/her functional alternative belief (FAB) after you and the adolescent have processed it in session. When the adolescent is in a deep stage of relaxation and in his/her safe place, you can lead the youth in the following guided imagery:

Find yourself in your very special and safe place—the most peaceful and special place in the world for you. Imagine being here and brighten up the scene and add all the details. I will be silent for a moment, as you do this. (PAUSE.) Now repeat the functional belief that you worked out with your therapist…just say the belief to yourself in your safe place. (PAUSE.) Stay in this safe place and slowly remember that you can move on in your life with all of yourself…feel the warmth and safety show you that you are really better than the sum of your life's experiences and you will move forward with your life…Breathe and allow yourself to relax for a moment…

Through guided imagery, you can teach the adolescent to determine the location of his/her perceptions on the fear continuum, to help overcome negative emotions such as fear, anger, and anxiety. This helps the adolescent understand and manage feelings more constructively. However, you would proceed after a thorough discussion of the fear(s) and only when you are certain that the adolescent is ready. For example, as explained above, when the adolescent is in a deep stage of relaxation and in his/her safe place in a guided imagery exercise, you can incorporate the following:

Get into a safe place, noticing your breathing. Now think back to the recent upsetting thing you're focusing on. Visualize what you were thinking and feeling prior to, and then during, the experience. On the 1 to 10 scale, how intense were you feeling? Do you remember how your breathing changed when you were upset? Was it shallow, quick? Now that you're relaxed, and breathing deeply, visualize your fear and anxiety. Continue to feel your breath and notice how when you breathe deeply, your thoughts are more clear, without any fear or anxiety. Now visualize yourself feeling relaxed and calm during a similar situation. The next time you are faced with a tense situation, you will remember how good it felt to be relaxed and in control. Remember these feelings…

Again, remember that the depth or intensity of the guided imagery has to be congruent with the youth's progress in the rest of the MDT process. The clinician needs to very carefully determine where the adolescent is on the therapeutic continuum to determine which mindfulness exercises are indicated. What is effective with one adolescent may not be effective with another.

Summary

Mindfulness enhances the adolescent's awareness of present experiences and the acceptance of self —crucial elements in the MDT process. It helps the adolescent learn to emotionally and cognitively defuse the strength of opposition and resistance to treatment and often to life in general. Overall, mindfulness is the context for the practice of MDT; therefore, as we repeatedly mention, the clinician needs to personally practice mindfulness in order to effectively incorporate it into MDT treatment. The next chapter explores MDT treatment of externalizing disorders, including how to work with your adolescent client and his/her family or caregivers in order to generalize MDT skills to the home and school environments.

Chapter 12

MDT Treatment of Externalizing Disorders

I n chapter 10, we discussed implementing MDT with adolescents to address internalizing disorders such as anxiety and depression, and in chapter 11 we practiced mindfulness exercises. This chapter addresses the use of MDT to manage behaviors characteristic of externalizing disorders, such as oppositional defiant disorder and conduct disorder. The constellation of aberrant behaviors presented by adolescents with these disorders can range from aggression, to disruptive and/or impulsive behaviors, to antisocial acts, to sometimes even criminal activity. We believe that untreated or mistreated fear and avoidance-based internalizing disorders are often the source of these behaviors. In other words, externalizing disorders are external manifestations of internally motivated fears. Adolescent self-management, as well as parent/caregiver collaboration and support, are important components in the generalization, implementation, and maintenance of functional behaviors in the MDT treatment of externalizing disorders. In the next few pages, we discuss the application of MDT in environments outside of the clinician's office. First, we begin with a discussion of the continuum scales.

Continuum Scales

The MDT Continuum Scales provide the adolescent and the clinician with a barometer of the therapeutic progress. There are five continuum scales addressing the most typical recurrent issues or areas in the treatment of angry, aggressive, and oppositional adolescents within MDT methodology. They are: Continuum of Anger, Continuum of Anticipated Fears, Continuum of Perception of Fears, Continuum of Physiological Responses, and Continuum of Trust. The continuums are quick and easy to use and they provide a concrete measure as well as facilitate the VCR component. Let's briefly describe each one.

- **Continuum of Anger** measures the adolescent's emotional dysregulation relevant to the perception of anger.

- **Continuum of Anticipated Fears** measures the cognitive processing of anxiety and fear associated with an anticipated event.

- **Continuum of Perception of Fears** measures the reactivity of a youth's perception associated with an "at risk" self-dysregulation.

- **Continuum of Physiological Responses** measures the youth's physiological responses to fear, danger, and stress.

- **Continuum of Trust** measures the levels of trust between the youth and the clinician or other persons.

The continuums are scales of 1 to 10, with a score of 1 being the lowest and a score of 10 the highest. Although they can be administered verbally, we suggest that whenever possible you complete them on paper. Having them in a written format allows the clinician and the adolescent to review them as needed for emerging patterns in the youth's behavioral and emotional changes. This visual record can also be useful later on in treatment when, for example, there is a functional behavioral lapse, and a record of positive change could be helpful in getting the youth back on track. The continuum scales are self-explanatory. They consist of two parts, typically a pretest and a posttest, with the posttest occurring at the clinician's office. For example, the youth completes the Continuum of Anticipated Fears prior to the challenging event and then again after the event in session with the clinician. The scales allow the adolescent and the clinician to concretely measure presented behavior, creating a reference point for evaluating future actions. They are especially useful for the clinician in the redirection phase of the validation, clarification, and redirection (VCR).

Continuum of Anger (Adolescent only)

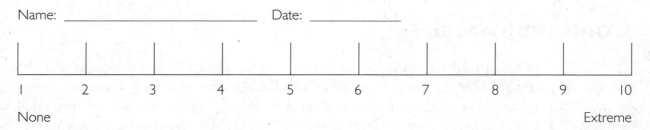

Name: _____   Date: _____

| | | | | | | | | |
| 1 | 2 | 3 | 4 | 5 | 6 | 7 | 8 | 9 | 10 |

None   Extreme

Adolescent Rates with Therapist

Name: _____   Date: _____

1	2	3	4	5	6	7	8	9	10

None   Extreme

****

Continuum of Trust

Name: _____   Date: _____

High Trust Person's Name: _____

1	2	3	4	5	6	7	8	9	10

None   Extreme

Most-Trusted Person's Name: _____

1	2	3	4	5	6	7	8	9	10

None   Extreme

Continuum of Anticipated Fears

Name: _____   Date: _____

Anticipated Experience: _____

Date of Anticipated Experience: _____

Your feeling(s) when you think of anticipated experience: _____

Prior to Experience

Name: _____   Date: _____

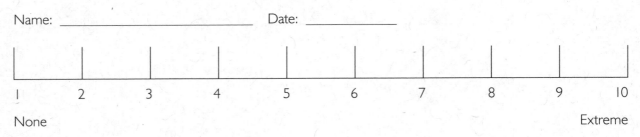

| | | | | | | | | | |
|1|2|3|4|5|6|7|8|9|10|

None   Extreme

After Experience – Adolescent Re-Rate with Therapist

Name: _____   Date: _____

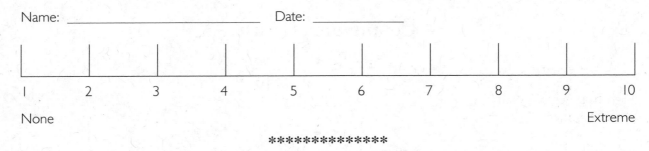

| | | | | | | | | | |
|1|2|3|4|5|6|7|8|9|10|

None   Extreme

****

Continuum of Perception of Fears

Name: _____   Date: _____

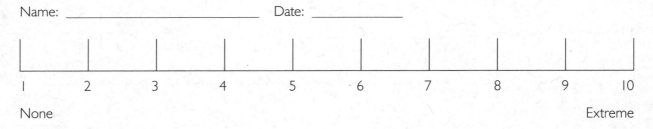

| | | | | | | | | | |
|1|2|3|4|5|6|7|8|9|10|

None   Extreme

Real Time Adolescent Rates with Therapist

Name: _____   Date: _____

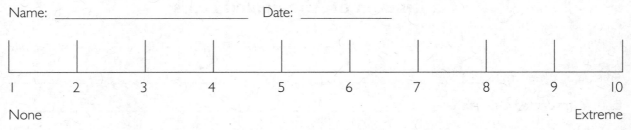

| | | | | | | | | | |
|1|2|3|4|5|6|7|8|9|10|

None   Extreme

****

Continuum of Physiological Responses

Rate your physiological response inside your body.

Name: _____   Date: _____

Identify your internal response. _____

Where do you notice a change in your body inside, when angry or afraid?_____

What kind of change do you notice in your body?_____

1	2	3	4	5	6	7	8	9	10

None   Extreme

Continuum of Physiological Responses Follow-up

After relaxation training, re-rate your physiological response with therapist.

Name: _____   Date: _____

Identify your internal response. _____

Where do you notice a change in your body inside, when angry or afraid?_____

What kind of change do you notice in your body?_____

1	2	3	4	5	6	7	8	9	10

None   Extreme

© 2009 Jack A. Apsche, EdD, ABPP

Along with the continuum scales, the adolescent employs a variety of MDT techniques to self-manage his/her externalized behaviors.

Adolescent Self-Management

As discussed throughout this book, the emotional and behavioral struggle experienced by opposi-tional, angry, and/or aggressive adolescents often originates from internalizing disorders. Through collaboration between the clinician and the adolescent, MDT efficiently addresses the youth's underlying fears, avoids, and beliefs to reduce the source and/or function of the problem behavior. This clinician/adolescent collaborative process is a twofold learning process for the adolescent to be able to balance beliefs. First, the adolescent endorses his/her compound core beliefs. Second, the adolescent adapts a functional or balanced belief by acknowledging the possibility of there being a different perspective or experience that is congruent with the functional alternative belief. The next step for the adolescent is to address these endorsed beliefs through self-management when applying MDT in his/her real-life environment. Mindfulness and acceptance are the initial keys to the self-management process.

Mindfulness and Acceptance

MDT trains the youth to "take a break" and do a breathing mindfulness exercise when he/she becomes aware of a negative change in mood, level of anger, or psychological response to cues in life. This break stops the escalation of dysfunctional reactions and provides the opportunity to defuse cognitive and behavioral negativity, allowing the adolescent to be more in control of himself/herself. Through this process, the adolescent implements the following sequence of MDT skills:

- Breathing mindfulness

- Emotional defusion

- Cognitive defusion

- Acceptance

- Balance belief into functional alternative belief

In this manner, the adolescent self-regulates, emotionally and physically. More specifically, the youth first locates the particular area(s) of physical tension and/or painful or negative thought(s), and then practices mindfulness, defusion, and acceptance exercises. The following scenario of an adolescent and a parent having a discussion about the youth's tardiness to school illustrates the process.

- The adolescent notices his/her level of anxiety increasing when speaking to the parent about being late to school.

- The adolescent figuratively steps back, takes a breath, and notices how he/she is breathing and proceeds to do a basic breathing exercise.

- The adolescent checks out himself/herself for angry and anxious feelings.

- He/she identifies these feelings and then cognitively and emotionally self-defuses. In other words, the youth allows himself/herself to experience the feeling(s) in the moment until he/she can separate from the pain. The adolescent can also defuse negative and anxious thoughts until the thoughts are devoid of powerful emotions.

- The adolescent moves to accepting that he/she is all right and can accept pain or anger in the moment.

By defusing cognitively and emotionally, the youth is able to balance beliefs as he/she regains cognitive and emotional regulation. Establishing this self-control allows the youth to, at a later time, calmly discuss his/her behavior (lateness) with the parent. The adolescent can also use the Conglomerate of Beliefs and Behaviors (COBB) to balance beliefs in challenging situations.

Conglomerate of Beliefs and Behaviors

In chapter 8, we introduced the COBB as a living document that stays with the adolescent throughout treatment. The COBB is essentially the scorecard for the adolescent's compound core beliefs and corresponding behaviors. Its function is to identify the adolescent's beliefs that activate the problematic behaviors. The adolescent can use the COBB independently of the clinician, parents, or caregivers, to balance beliefs. Here's a summary of the process. First, the adolescent identifies the problem behavior. Then, using the COBB, the youth makes the connection between the problem behavior and the activated compound core belief. Next, the adolescent balances the identified belief by turning it into a functional alternative belief (FAB). For example, the belief "Anything is better than feeling unpleasant" may activate in an adolescent behaviors such as smoking marijuana, avoiding contact with painful emotions, isolating from others, or engaging in parasuicidal gestures. Through MDT treatment, the adolescent learns to become aware when, for example, he/she begins to physically or emotionally isolate from others. Through the use of the COBB, he/she can then relate the act of isolating from others to the belief "Anything is better than feeling unpleasant." Consequently, the youth can then turn this compound core belief into a FAB. That is, the adolescent can review the original, precipitating belief and substitute it with the FAB, "I have felt bad before and I did okay." This change in perspective may also later be reflected by the adolescent's engaging in more positive social activity, getting along at home, and continuing the MDT treatment plan. Parents or caregivers can also use the COBB, along with other MDT techniques, to help the adolescent balance beliefs, as described in the next section.

Parent or Caregiver Collaboration

Parent and caregiver collaboration is an integral component of MDT treatment in order to fully support and encourage the youth to engage in functional alternative behaviors at home and other environments. In other words, significant figures in the adolescent's life need to be well-versed in the language of MDT; for example, mindfulness, COBB, and VCR of the FAB. The implementation of MDT skills outside of individual sessions follows the same methodology that the clinician uses in individual therapy. There are instances in which family MDT treatment is also recommended; however, as previously indicated, an in-depth look at family MDT is beyond the scope of this book. To effectively collaborate in the adolescent's treatment, the parent/caregiver needs to actually have a copy of the COBB as reference (with the adolescent's knowledge and agreement, of course). In the following section, we provide examples of how a parent/caregiver can incorporate MDT skills to help the adolescent manage problematic behaviors.

MDT Skills Application

Let's take, for example, an angry and aggressive female adolescent who gets into verbal and physical altercations with her peers. One fear that activates this particular behavior in the adolescent is feeling that "Something is wrong with me." Consequently, the youth then avoids being vulnerable and honest with her emotions because the fear activates the belief "Whenever I feel, it is horrible." Once this activation begins, a chain reaction occurs. In other words, the adolescent's fears and avoidance are subsequently activated by the belief. This fear/avoidance activation, in turn, results in the youth's heightened physiological and emotional arousal leading to verbal and physical fights with peers.

When the parent/caregiver is familiar with MDT and notices that the adolescent's behavior is off-balance, he/she can implement a VCR intervention to help the youth balance her FAB. For instance, the parent/caregiver can say at the appropriate times:

Validation: You have felt like you were getting hyped before and have been able to interrupt yourself with your breathing and mindfulness exercises.

Clarification: So can we or you practice it in the moment like you have done before?

Redirection: Is it possible that in this moment you can sit back and let yourself experience your painful feelings and anger and be okay? On a scale of 1 to 10, how much do you believe you can be okay in the moment with your feelings? You just successfully experienced your unpleasant feelings and you are okay!

Such use of VCR by the parent/caregiver helps the adolescent be able to cognitively access the FAB. The next sample dialogue demonstrates how a parent can guide the adolescent to balance beliefs through the use of the COBB and VCR.

Parent: So, Mark, you have been isolating yourself in your room and not communicating your feelings much.

Adolescent: Yeah, I have been feeling off.

Parent: What belief do you think is related to that behavior? Let's look at your COBB.

Adolescent: Anything is better than feeling like crap.

Parent: Yes, I agree. Can I ask you something?

Adolescent: Yes, I know, the last time I felt like that I did okay.

Parent: And you worked on it with your therapist, right?

Adolescent: Yeah, I know, 6 or 7 out of 10.

Parent: So, you could feel bad and be okay. How about right now in this moment? Can you feel bad right now and know you will deal with it okay?

Adolescent: Yeah, I think so.

Parent: Do you want to do some breathing exercises?

Adolescent: Yeah, but alone. Okay?

Parent: Okay.

Adolescent: [*Begins to work on math.*]

Parent: [*Leaving.*] I'll check in later.

In the previous example, the adolescent and the parent used the same frame of reference: the COBB, VCR of the FAB, and mindfulness. The adolescent in this scenario was able to engage in a fairly calm conversation with the parent in order to be redirected. However, sometimes, the adolescent's emotional dysregulation needs to be addressed first before any cognitive work can be successful; for example, in the case of escalating anger that may lead to aggression. In such a scenario, the parental approach may be to guide the adolescent to initiate mindfulness prior to the VCR of the FAB, as shown in this next dialogue:

Parent: I've noticed that you've been extremely tense and irritable recently.

Adolescent: So?

Parent: I understand that you've been feeling something and it seems to be unsettling you.

Adolescent: Yeah.

Parent: So, instead of talking, let's just practice some breathing, either together or alone. See if it will help?

Adolescent: I don't feel like it.

Parent: Okay, but it has helped me and we've done this together. It may be helpful.

Adolescent: Okay, breathing.

Parent: Can you lead us in breathing so we do it your way?

Adolescent: Okay. [*Starts somewhat reluctantly.*] Take a breath through your mouth, and then hold it a second then exhale through your nose. Notice the seconds between your inhale and exhale. Clear your mind; just notice the peace. Inhale…Exhale.

(*They do five minutes of breathing.*)

Adolescent: Okay, open your eyes when you're comfortable.

Parent: I feel peaceful. How about you?

Adolescent: Yes, I can feel myself centered.

Parent: What belief was activating your emotions?

Adolescent: Anything is better than feeling unpleasant.

Parent: Okay, where were your unpleasant feelings?

Adolescent: In my chest. It was heavy.

Parent: So, let's sit and let yourself know that you've felt these feelings before and were okay.

Adolescent: I know.

Parent: Any thoughts?

Adolescent: I can achieve anything. I am worthy. I know I can be okay with unpleasant feelings. I just do my breathing and mindfulness and accept myself and it seems okay.

Parent: You can do this with me or on your own. You've done so great with your work on yourself.

Adolescent: Yeah, thanks.

Parent: This is so much better than fighting and yelling. Great work! [*Smiles at adolescent.*]

In the above situation, the use of mindfulness allowed the adolescent to gain control of his emotions in order to ultimately balance his beliefs. Notice that the parent participated fully in the breathing exercise, which regulates the parent's own emotions and allows him/her to interact with the adolescent in a calm manner. But what happens if the adolescent reverts to previous aberrant behaviors?

Lapses in Behavior

If the adolescent lapses back into angry or aggressive behaviors, first, it is important to look at the problem or lapse as a temporary setback, not a permanent regression or treatment failure. In fact, reverting to previous negative behaviors at one time or another is somewhat expected in treatment. Remember that the problems experienced by severely oppositional, angry, and aggressive adolescents most likely developed as a result of years of abuse, neglect, or other dysfunctional situations or environments. Therefore, each adolescent's treatment pathway is unique in its intensity, direction, and duration.

Second, when addressing lapses to previously learned negative behavior, besides noting the adolescent's transgressions, it is important to take an honest look at a variety of factors that may also have influenced the youth. For example, how did you approach the youth with your VCR? Is the adolescent practicing mindfulness and breathing exercises? Has a parent, caregiver, or staff member slipped back into a nonreinforcing negative, abusive, or demanding verbal practice style rather than a VCR approach? What belief or beliefs were activated in the adolescent during the lapse? Is there a need to review the case conceptualization to identify any additional beliefs and fears that were not previously recognized? The responses to these questions can guide you in determining the next step of treatment.

Discuss with the youth the behavioral lapse. Listen to his/her story. You and the adolescent may want to conduct a situational analysis to understand what happened. Together you can reexamine the COBB and the TFAB worksheet, or it may be useful to review some of the mindfulness exercises. As you and the adolescent begin to reframe the dysfunctional behavior into a FAB, go over any past continuum scales that may provide a record of past success for the adolescent. Remember that whenever a human being experiences pressure or fear, he/she might revert to previous coping behaviors—whether functional or dysfunctional. Through MDT, the clinician can provide validation, clarification, and redirection to the adolescent in order to make an aversive situation a positive learning and growth opportunity.

Summary

This chapter has moved MDT from a psychotherapy to a living, breathing intervention for adolescents. It also engages parents/caregivers in the creation of a mindful relationship with the adolescent and the incorporation of mindfulness in their own lives as well. Much of MDT can be generalized throughout adolescence and into adulthood to maintain balance and harmony throughout life. We suggest you review the steps presented in this chapter until you are comfortable and feel competent to bring the parent or caregiver into the MDT session. Remember, you also have a responsibility to collaborate with the adolescent and teach the steps to self-management using MDT. You have the difficult task to get the parents or caregivers to participate and achieve a level of familiarity with the practice of mindfulness and the process of validation, clarification, and redirection of the functional alternative belief. This all rests with your level of comfort and practice of these methodologies. Please never just "wing it" or "fly by the seat of your pants." Over the years, we have witnessed many well-intentioned clinicians who believe they can use the force of their will or their charisma to mitigate their lack of preparation and training. The end result is always the same; they cannot help the adolescent and his/her family. To work with difficult, oppositional, and aggressive adolescents can be a difficult task, and to not prepare for a session with a methodology that is effective is only going to make life more difficult for the adolescent, the family, and yourself. In our conclusion we provide some final recommendations for treating adolescents with MDT.

Conclusion

We hope that by reading this book you have discovered the value of MDT methodology and are ready to join us in finding how effective it can be in adolescent treatment. If you are an ACT-trained therapist, you will find learning MDT is an easy transition for you. If you are working with an adolescent who is not responding well to other treatment modalities, we suggest you use MDT. Remember, MDT has been successfully implemented with some very difficult oppositional, angry, and aggressive adolescents who have even been labeled by various therapists and systems of care as dangerous, conduct disordered youths, or impossible to treat oppositional, angry adolescents.

There are additional tools, which will be available soon, that can advance your proficiency in MDT in your work with adolescents. These MDT resources include an adolescent client manual, a mindfulness manual, and a family assessment and treatment manual. We also recommend that you attend an MDT workshop to continue your training.

We are often asked whether MDT is effective with other populations, such as adolescents with borderline personality or substance abuse disorders, or even with adults. The consistent response, so far, is that we cannot confirm that MDT will or will not be effective with these populations because we have no final MDT research data with these populations—yet. However, we are indeed beginning to study the efficacy of MDT on populations beyond sexual offenders and angry, aggressive, and oppositional adolescents. Recently, several colleagues and I (J. Apsche) completed a study examining the use of MDT in the treatment of adolescent males with substance abuse and comorbid mental health disorders. Preliminary results suggest that MDT may have a positive effect in treating this particular subset of youths (Apsche, 2011).

We believe that MDT is a vibrant and growing therapeutic methodology that may be useful with many yet undetermined populations, which future applications, research, and development will identify. We invite you to be a part of this growth in both treatment and research. Lastly, it has been a wonderful and exhilarating experience writing this book to offer you what we believe is an effective methodology for angry, aggressive, and oppositional adolescents. We look forward to your feedback and success in treating adolescents with MDT.

Appendix A

Typology Survey

TYPOLOGY SURVEY

I. Identifying Information
1. Client Name:
2. Date of Birth/Age:
3. Ethnicity:
4. Date:

	Client Interview	Parent/Guardian	Collateral Information
II. Family Information			
1. Briefly describe each member of the family (please indicate who resides with the client). Include any children with their ages and gender.			
2. Indicate all the places that the client has lived in his life.			
3. Where does the client plan to live after leaving home?			
4. Describe relationship of the client's parents (include marital status).			
5. Describe relationship between client and mother/ guardian.			
6. Describe relationship between client and father/ guardian.			
7. Describe what the client/ parent/ guardian would like to see change about their relationship.			
8. Describe relationship between client and siblings.			
9. What is the best thing and worst thing mother/guardian has ever done for/to the client?	Best: Worst:	Best: Worst:	Best: Worst:

10. What is the best thing and worst thing father/guardian has ever done for/to the client?	Best: Worst:	Best: Worst:	Best: Worst:
11. Is there anyone in client's family he does not like to be with? Who and Why?			
12. Indicate whom the client talks to when he/she feels worried, sad, or scared.			
13. Any other relevant information about family?			

	Client Interview	Parent/Guardian	Collateral Information
III. Substance Abuse History			
1. What drugs/alcohol have you used?			
2. If you have used, how often, and for how long?			
3. Do you believe your use of drugs/alcohol has affected your ability to function?			
4. Referral to chemical dependency counselor?			

	Client Interview	Parent/ Guardian	Collateral Information
IV. Medical			
1. Has the client been to the hospital? If so, explain.			
2. Is the client taking any medication? If so, for what reason?			
3. Does the client have a history of childhood head trauma, hits to the head, or central nervous system trauma?			
4. Is there history of intrauterine drug or alcohol usage? Did mother use any substances prior to the birth of the child?			

	Client Interview	Parent/ Guardian	Collateral Information
V. Educational			
1. What grade is the client in? Special education?			
2. How is the client doing in school?			
3. What are the client's academic goals? (GED, diploma, college, technical school, etc.)			
4. Has the client held a job? If so, when and where?			
5. Describe any previous training or preparation for vocational training and/or independent living.			

	Client Interview	Parent/ Guardian	Collateral Information
VI. Emotional			
1. What is your usual mood like? (If negative, ask: When was it last good)			
2. What do you do when you are sad?			
3. Suicidal ideation - Have you ever thought of hurting yourself? How? If yes, when was the last time you felt this way? Please explain circumstances.			
4. Have you ever tried to hurt yourself in any way? (when, how, where, what happened)			
5. Are there any unpleasant memories that keep coming back to you? What are they?			

6. How have you been sleeping? Do you experience any of the following: trouble falling asleep; trouble waking in the morning; waking in the middle of the night; tiredness during the day; nightmares			
7. Has your interest in food increased or decreased? Have you gained or lost weight recently?			
8. Is there a history of bedwetting? Describe.			
9. Does the client have a history of fire setting? Describe.			
10. Have you ever run away from home or other residence? If yes, please explain?			
11. Describe the client's aberrant behaviors.			
12. Has the client ever been in counseling before? If so, describe.			
13. Has the client ever been hospitalized? If so, for what and when?			
14. Has the client ever been in another treatment program? If so, for what and when?			
15. What does the client usually do when he/she gets really upset or angry?			
16. Has the client ever intentionally harmed animals?			
17. Has the client ever destroyed things or hit anyone in anger? If so, tell me about it.			
18. Homicidal ideation - Has the client ever been so mad that he/she wanted to really hurt or kill someone else? If so, when, how, where, why.			

VII. Physiological			
1. Describe an incident where the client was angry or upset.			
2. Ask the client for descriptions of specific physiological responses. Describe what "my face is red," "my blood boils," clenched fists, teeth and jaws feel like and what do these feelings mean? Take your time and ask about breathing; all responses. Rank in order the physiological responses and how the client responds to them. Rank from first physiological response to final physiological response. (Remember, muscle tightened, stomach tightened, etc.)	Examples: Gritting teeth Clenching fists Sweating Face and arms flush Redness of face Veins bulge Jittery Shaking Crying Frowning Heart rate increases Shortness of breath Loss or change in vocal pitch Burning in chest Stomach/ intestinal pains Cramping Exhaustion/ fatigue Nervous twitching Raised voice	Client's physiological responses	Ranked physiological responses
	Client Interview	Parent/ Guardian	Collateral Information

VIII. Interpersonal Relationships/Social History			
1. What did you typically do in the afternoons after school and on the weekends?			
2. What kinds of things do you do for fun?			
3. How old were you when you had your first sexual experience?			
4. Sexual Orientation: (Heterosexual, Homosexual, Bisexual, Unsure)			
5. How many sexual partners have you had?			
6. What type of birth control did you use?			
7. Has any physical or emotional maltreatment occurred in any of your social relationships? If yes, please explain.			
8. Has the client engaged in any sexual behaviors? If so, has he/she received any type of previous treatment?			

IX. Behavioral Data

Problem Behavior

		Victim's name/ relationship	Client's age	Victim's age	# of incidents	Describe the behavior	How did the client get the victim to go along?	How did the client get caught?	What are the related charges?
1	Client interview:								
	Parent/guardian:								
	Collateral Information:								
2	Client interview:								
	Parent/guardian:								
	Collateral Information:								
3	Client interview:								
	Parent/guardian:								
	Collateral Information:								
4	Client interview:								

	Parent/guardian:							
	Collateral Information:							
5	Client interview:							
	Parent/guardian:							
	Collateral Information:							
6	Client interview:							
	Parent/guardian:							
	Collateral Information:							
7	Client interview:							
	Parent/guardian:							
	Collateral Information:							
Total number of victims:			Total number of offenses (incidents):			Total number of charges:		

X. History of Physical and Sexual Abuse:

History of Physical Abuse

		Perpetrator's name/ relationship	Client's age at onset	Duration	Perp's age	# of incidents	Describe the abuse (hitting, use objects, burning, etc.)	How did the perpetrator get the client to go along?	How and when was it discovered (client's age at the time of the discovery)?	What was done about the abuse when it was discovered?	Has the abuse been reported?	Outcome of reporting
1	Client interview:											
	Parent/ guardian:											
	Collateral Information:											
2	Client interview:											
	Parent/ guardian:											
	Collateral Information:											
3	Client interview:											
	Parent/ guardian:											

Collateral Information:											
4 Client interview:											
Parent/ guardian:											
Collateral Information:											
5 Client interview:											
Parent/ guardian:											
Collateral Information:											

Is there any other relevant information regarding history of physical abuse?

History of Sexual Abuse

		Perpetrator's name/ relationship	Client's age at onset	Duration	Perp's age	# of incidents	Describe the abuse (Oral, anal, vaginal, fondling, animal, digital penetration, stalking, telephone scatalogia, flashing, frottage, combination, etc.).	How did the perpetrator get the client to go along?	How and when was it discovered (client's age at the time of the discovery)?	What was done about the abuse when it was discovered?	Has the abuse been reported?	Outcome of reporting
1	Client interview:											
	Parent/ guardian:											
	Collateral Information:											
2	Client interview:											
	Parent/ guardian:											
	Collateral Information:											

3	Client interview:										
	Parent/ guardian:										
	Collateral Information:										
4	Client interview:										
	Parent/ guardian:										
	Collateral Information:										
5	Client interview:										
	Parent/ guardian:										
	Collateral Information:										

Is there any other relevant information regarding history of sexual abuse?

XI. History of Other Abuse	Client Interview	Parent/ Guardian	Collateral Information
Emotional Abuse Client's history of emotional abuse.			
1. Indicate who the perpetrator is; include relationship to client (family member, an individual known to the family, stranger).			
2. Age of onset, duration.			
3. Describe the abuse.			
4. How and when was the emotional abuse discovered? (include the client's age at the time of the discovery)			
5. What was done about the abuse when it was discovered?			
6. Has the emotional abuse been reported? If so, what was the outcome?			
7. Is there any suggestion that the client was subjected to emotional invalidation as a child or adolescent by primary caregiver?			
Neglect			
8. Describe any neglect the client has experienced (lack of shelter, food, clothing, love, environmental deprivation, etc.). Include the length of time the neglect was suffered.			
9. Describe the environment the client was raised in. Include SES (socioeconomic status)			
10. Was either parent frequently away or out of the home at any time in the client's life? If yes, please explain.			
Other Trauma			
11. Describe any other trauma the client has experienced, e.g., witness the death of someone, or have their life threatened? Severity?			

	Client Interview	Parent/ Guardian	Collateral Information
12. Age of onset, frequency.			
13. Has the client lost contact with anyone special to him/her (e.g., death, imprisonment, etc.)?			
14. Indicate any physical violence the client has ever witnessed between family members? Please explain.			
15. Has the client ever witnessed any violence? Describe.			
16. Describe family stresses at this time (e.g., financial, marital difficulties, etc.)			
17. Indicate if the client has been involved in a gang or crew in his neighborhood.			
18. Is there a history of group (neighborhood) influence on his behavior? Give details.			
19. What "survival skills" did the client need to survive in home environment?			

XII. Expectations of Treatment	Client Interview	Parent/ Guardian	Collateral Information
1. What would the client like to do differently when he is discharged?			
2. What are some goals the client has for the next year?			
3. Willingness and motivation to be involved in family therapy sessions.			
4. If the client could change anything about him/herself, what would he/she change?			

© 2005 Jack A. Apsche, EdD, ABPP

Appendix B

Your Turn Responses
(Chapter 10)

Response Key

Mindfulness (M)

Emotional Defusion (ED)

Cognitive Defusion (CD)

Acceptance (A)

Validation, clarification and redirection of the functional alternative belief (VCR of the FAB)

Breathing Mindfulness (BM)

Validation (V)

> *Therapist:* It seems that you had a rough weekend, according to your mother.
>
> *Adolescent:* She exaggerates sometimes.
>
> *Therapist:* Did she this time?
>
> *Adolescent:* Well, I did cut myself and smoke some weed.
>
> *Therapist:* You know, I think we should focus on you now in this moment…so can we do some mindfulness breathing? (M)

Adolescent: I am not into it right now. It won't work. (M)

Therapist: Since you are breathing anyway, why not breathe together? (M)

Adolescent: Okay, okay.

Therapist: Inhale through your mouth and exhale through your nose. Notice the brief nano-second that you are not breathing, Let yourself experience that brief moment of peace and as you exhale, silently say "One." Good. Inhale. Experience a moment of peace. Exhale to "One." (M)

[The exercise was continued for about 4 minutes with client]

Therapist: Okay, now what do you notice that you are feeling emotionally? (ED)

Adolescent: Nothing—I am empty and numb. (ED)

Therapist: Can you tell me where your emptiness is in your body? (ED)

Adolescent: [*Points to her chest and heart.*] (ED)

Therapist: Describe the feeling of emptiness and numbness in your chest and heart. (ED)

Adolescent: It is like it is cold and I am feeling nothing there. (ED)

Therapist: As you look deeper in your heart and chest, what might you feel behind your emptiness? (ED)

Adolescent: You mean the pain and deep ache like my heart is going to blow up? (ED)

Therapist: Yes, that's it. Can you let yourself go behind the numbness and feel that pain right here? (ED)

Adolescent: [*Begins to weep and is clearly experiencing painful emotions.*] (ED)

Therapist: Can you tell me some of the painful thoughts that are attached to these painful feelings? (CD)

Adolescent: I am shit, nothing, worthless. Life is a waste and no one gives a fuck about me. (CD)

Therapist: Good, but what do all these words really mean? They are just words. (CD)

Adolescent: Maybe so, but they hurt. (CD)

Therapist: Look at the word "worthless." Let's repeat it together 10 times. "Worthless, worthless, worthless…" (CD)

Adolescent: [Repeats "worthless" 10 times with therapist.] (CD)

Therapist: It sounds silly, but it *is* silly in a way, because it is only a word. Nothing but a word. You have all these emotions attached to this word. (CD)

Adolescent: Okay, so? (CD)

Therapist: So, you were able to sit and experience your painful emotions and your painful thoughts and you are still here and okay, right?

Adolescent: Yes, but I am feeling anxious. (A)

Therapist: Okay. You now have experienced these painful thoughts and feelings and are only a little anxious. Right? (A)

Adolescent: Yes. (A)

Therapist: You can decide that if you experience these painful feelings or thoughts, you can survive. But then, these feelings might come and go throughout your life. Can you accept that might be true? (A)

Adolescent: I don't like it, but I can accept it. (A)

Therapist: So, are you ready to move forward with your life together with your painful feelings and emotions, right now? (A)

Adolescent: It isn't easy, but I will try. (A)

Therapist: Is that a yes? (A)

Adolescent: Yes. (A)

Therapist: Good. What belief is activating and setting off these painful thoughts and emotions? (VCR)

Adolescent: I can't deal with unpleasant feelings, and anything is better than feeling unpleasant or feeling pain. (VCR)

Therapist: You endorsed those beliefs with a "4" or "Always," correct? (VCR)

Adolescent: Yes. (VCR)

Therapist: You realize that right here today, you were able to deal with your painful thoughts and emotions and were okay? (VCR)

Adolescent: Yes, but I still feel my heart pounding.

Therapist: That's okay. But you now know that there are times, like right here and right now, that you can deal with your pain. So, on a scale of 1 to 10, how much do you think that it is possible for you to deal with your painful beliefs? (VCR)

Adolescent: Around a 5 or so. (VCR)

Therapist: Great. So, 50 percent of the time, you can experience these painful feelings and thoughts and be okay with them? (VCR)

Adolescent: Yes, I think I can. (VCR)

Therapist: That is amazing! You have found a possible alternative, 50 percent of the time, to cutting or smoking weed. (VCR)

Adolescent: That's what I said. (VCR)

Therapist: Great work. Can we finish our session today with a breathing exercise? (BM)

Adolescent: Yes, I want to do that. (BM)

[The same breathing mindfulness exercise from the beginning of the session is repeated for five minutes to alleviate her anxiety and complete the session.] (BM)

Therapist: You feeling okay now?

Adolescent: Yes, better.

Therapist: On a scale of 1 to 10, where is your anxiety? (V)

Adolescent: Only a 1.5. (V)

Therapist: Okay, great work! (V)

References

Achenbach, T. M. (1991). *Integrative guide to the 1991 CBCL/4-18, YSR and TRF Profiles.* Burlington, VT: University of Vermont.

American Psychiatric Association. (2000). *Diagnostic and statistical manual of mental disorders* (4th ed., text rev.). Washington, DC: Author.

Alford, B. A., & Beck, A. T. (1997). *The integrative power of cognitive therapy.* New York: Guilford Press.

Apsche, J. A. (2010). *Mode deactivation therapy: The complete guidebook for clinicians.* Unpublished manuscript.

Apsche, J. A. (2011). *Case study of an adolescent with poly substance abuse issues.* Manuscript submitted for publication.

Apsche, J. A., & Bass, C. K. (2006). A treatment study of mode deactivation therapy in an outpatient community setting. *International Journal of Behavioral Consultation and Therapy, 2,* 85–93.

Apsche, J. A., & Bass, C. K. (2010). Treating physically and sexually aggressive adolescents and their families with mode deactivation therapy. In B. Schwartz (Ed.), *The sex offender* (Vol. 7). Kingston, NJ: Civic Research Institute.

Apsche, J. A., Bass, C. K., & DiMeo, L. (2010). Mode Deactivation Therapy (MDT) comprehensive meta-analysis. *Journal of Behavior Analysis of Offender and Victim Treatment and Protection, 2,* 171–182.

Apsche, J. A., Bass, C. K., & Houston, M.-A. (2007). Family MDT: vs. treatment as usual in a community setting. *International Journal of Behavioral Consultation and Therapy, 3,* 145–153.

Apsche, J. A., Bass, C. K., Jennings, J. L., Murphy, C. J., Hunter, J. A., & Siv, A. M. (2005). Empirical comparison of three treatments for adolescent males with physical and sexual aggression: Mode deactivation therapy, cognitive behavioral therapy and social skills training. *International Journal of Behavioral Consultation and Therapy, 1*, 101–113.

Apsche, J. A., Bass, C. K., Jennings, J. L., & Siv, A. M. (2005). A review and empirical comparison of two treatments for adolescent males with conduct and personality disorders: Mode deactivation therapy and cognitive behavior therapy. *International Journal of Behavioral Consultation and Therapy, 1*, 27–45.

Apsche, J. A., Bass, C. K., & Murphy, C. J. (2004). An empirical comparison of cognitive behavior therapy (CBT) and mode deactivation therapy (MDT) with adolescent males with conduct disorder and/or personality traits and sexually reactive behaviors. *Behavior Analyst Today, 5*, 359–371.

Apsche, J. A., Bass, C. K., & Siv, A. M. (2005). A review and empirical comparison of three treatments for adolescent males with conduct and personality disorder. *International Journal of Behavioral Consultation and Therapy, 1*, 312–322.

Apsche, J. A., Bass, C. K., & Siv, A. M. (2006). A treatment study of a suicidal adolescent with personality disorder or traits: Mode deactivation therapy as compared to treatment as usual. *International Journal of Behavioral Consultation and Therapy, 2*, 215–223.

Apsche, J. A., Bass, C. K., Siv, A. M., & Matteson, S. C. (2005). An empirical "real world" comparison of two treatments with aggressive adolescent males. *International Journal of Behavioral Consultation and Therapy, 1*, 239–251.

Apsche, J. A., Bass, C. K., Zeiter, S., & Houston, M. A. (2009). Family mode deactivation therapy in a residential setting: Treating adolescents with conduct disorder and multi-axial diagnosis. *International Journal of Behavioral Consultation and Therapy, 4*, 328–339.

Apsche, J. A., & DiMeo, L. (2010). Application of mode deactivation therapy to juvenile sex abusers. In S. Bengis & D. Prescott (Eds.), *Current applications: Strategies for working with sexually aggressive youth and youth with sexual behavior problems.* Holyoke, MA: Neari Press.

Apsche, J. A., Ward Bailey, S., & Evile, M. M. (2003). Mode deactivation therapy: A functionally based treatment, theoretical constructs. *Behavior Analyst Today, 3*(6), 455–459.

Apsche, J. A., & Ward, S. R. (2003). Mode deactivation therapy and cognitive behavior therapy: A description of treatment results for adolescents with personality beliefs, sexual offending and aggressive behaviors. *Behavior Analyst Today, 3*, 460–470.

Barlow, D. H. (2002). *Anxiety and its disorders: The nature and treatment of anxiety and panic* (2nd ed.). New York: Guilford Press.

Beck, A. T. (1996). Beyond belief: A theory of modes, personality and psychopathology. In P. M. Salkovaskis (Ed.), *Frontiers of cognitive therapy*. New York: Guilford Press.

Beck, A. T., Emery, G., & Greenberg, R. L. (1985). *Anxiety disorders and phobias: A cognitive perspective*. New York: Basic Books.

Beck, A. T., Freeman, A., & Associates. (1990). *Cognitive therapy of personality disorders*. New York: Guilford Press.

Berkowitz, L. (1990). On the formulation and regulation of anger and aggression: A cognitive-neoassociationistic analysis. *American Psychologist, 45*, 494–503.

Birmaher, B., Ryan, N. D., Williamson, D. E., Brent, D. A., Kaufman, J., Dahl, R. E., et al. (1996). Childhood and adolescent depression: A review of the past 10 years. Part I. *Journal of the American Academy of Child and Adolescent Psychiatry, 35*, 1427–1439.

Brent, D. A., Holder, D., Kolko, D., Birmaher, B., Baugher, M., Roth, C., et al. (1997). A clinical psychotherapy trial for adolescent depression comparing cognitive, family, and supportive treatments. *Archives of General Psychiatry, 54*, 877–885.

Brown, K., Atkins, M. S., Osbourne, M. L., & Milnamow, M. (1996). A revised teacher rating scale for reactive and proactive aggression. *Journal of Abnormal Child Psychology, 24*, 473–481.

Cartwright-Hatton, S., McNicol, K., & Doubleday, E. (2006). Anxiety in a neglected population: Prevalence of anxiety disorders in pre-adolescent children. *Clinical Psychology Review, 26*, 817–833.

Chamberlain, P. (2003). *Treating chronic juvenile offenders: Advances made through the Oregon multidimensional treatment foster care model*. Washington, DC: American Psychological Association.

Chorpita, B. F., & Barlow, D. H. (1998). The development of anxiety: The role of control in the early environment. *Psychological Bulletin, 124*, 3–21.

Clark, D. A., & Beck, A. T. (2010). *Cognitive therapy of anxiety disorders*. New York: Guilford Press.

Clarke, G. N., & DeBar, L. L. (2010). Group cognitive-behavioral treatment for adolescent depression. In J. R. Weisz & A. E. Kazdin (Eds.), *Evidence-based psychotherapies for children and adolescents*. New York: Guilford Press.

Cohen, J. A., Mannarino, A. P., & Deblinger, E. (2010). Trauma-focused cognitive-behavioral therapy for traumatized children. In J. R. Weisz & A. E. Kazdin (Eds.), *Evidence-based psychotherapies for children and adolescents*. New York: Guilford Press.

Dodge, K. A., & Coie, J. D. (1987). Social information processing factors in reactive and proactive aggression in children's peer groups. *Journal of Personality and Social Psychology, 53*, 1146–1158.

Dodge, K. D., Lochman, J. E., Harnish, J. D., Bates, J. E., & Pettit, G. S. (1997). Reactive and proactive aggression in school children and psychiatrically impaired chronically assaultive youth. *Journal of Abnormal Psychology, 106*, 37–51.

Dollard, J., Doob, L. W., Miller, N. E., Mowrer, O. H., & Sears, R. R. (1939). *Frustration and aggression.* New Haven, CT: Yale University Freer.

Dougher, M. J. (1994). The act of acceptance. In S. C. Hayes, N. Jacobsen, V. Follette, & M. J. Dougher (Eds.), *Acceptance and change: Content and context in psychotherapy.* Reno, NV: Context Press.

Forgatch, M. S., & Patterson, G. R. (2010). Parent management training-Oregon model: An intervention for antisocial behavior in children and adolescents. In J. R. Weisz & A. E. Kazdin (Eds.), *Evidence-based psychotherapies for children and adolescents.* New York: Guilford Press.

Greco, L. A., & Hayes, S. C. (2008). *Acceptance and mindfulness treatments for children and adolescents: A practitioner's guide.* Oakland, CA: New Harbinger.

Greene, R. W., & Ablon, J. S. (2006). *Treating explosive kids: The collaborative problem-solving approach.* New York: Guilford Press.

Hayes, S. C. (1994). Content, context, and the types of psychological acceptance. In S. C. Hayes, N. S. Jacobson, V. M. Follette, & M. J. Dougher (Eds.), *Acceptance and change: Content and context in psychotherapy.* Reno, NV: Context Press.

Hayes, S. C. (2004). Acceptance and commitment therapy, relational frame theory, and the third wave of behavioral and cognitive therapies. *Behavior Therapy, 35*, 639–665.

Hayes, S. C., Barnes-Holmes, D., & Roche, B. (Eds.). (2001). *Relational frame theory: A post-Skinnerian account of human language and cognition.* New York: Plenum Press.

Hayes, S. C., Strosahl, K., & Wilson, K. G. (1999). *Acceptance and commitment therapy: An experiential approach to behavior change.* New York: Guilford Press.

Hayes, S. C., Wilson, K. W., Gifford, E. V., Follette, V. M., & Strosahl, K. (1996). Experiential avoidance and behavioral disorders: A functional dimensional approach to diagnosis and treatment. *Journal of Consulting and Clinical Psychology, 64*, 1152–1168.

Henggeler, S. W. (1982). *Delinquency and adolescent psychopathology: A family-ecological systems approach.* Littleton, MA: John Wright-PSG.

Henggeler, S. W., Letourneau, E. J., Chapman, J. E., Borduin, C. M., Schewe, P. A., & McCart, M. R. (2009). Mediators of change for multisystemic therapy with juvenile sexual offenders. *Journal of the American Academy of Child and Adolescent Psychology, 77*, 451–462.

Henggeler, S. W., & Schaeffer, C. (2010). Treating serious antisocial behavior using multisystemic therapy. In J. R. Weisz & A. E. Kazdin (Eds.), *Evidence-based psychotherapies for children and adolescents*. New York: Guilford Press.

Henggeler, S. W., Schoenwald, S. K., Borduin, C. M., Rowland, M. D., & Cunningham, P. B. (2009). *Multisystemic therapy for antisocial behavior in children and adolescents* (2nd ed.). New York: Guilford Press.

Johnson, J. G., Cohen, P., Brown, J., Smailes, E. M., & Bernstein, D. P. (1999). Childhood maltreatment increases the risk for personality disorders during early childhood. *Archives of General Psychiatry, 56*, 600–608.

Johnson, J. G., Cohen, P., Smailes, E. M., Skodol, A. E., Brown, J., & Oldham, J. M. (2001). Childhood verbal abuse and risk for development of personality disorders. *Directions in Psychiatry: The Journal of Continuing Medical Education in Psychiatry, 14*, 171–187.

Johnson, J. G., Smailes, E. M., Cohen, P., Brown, J., & Bernstein, D. P. (2000). Associations between four types of childhood neglect and personality disorder symptoms during adolescence and early adulthood: Findings of a community based longitudinal study. *Journal of Personality Disorders, 14*, 171–187.

Kazdin, A. E. (2005). *Parent management training: Treatment for oppositional, aggressive, and antisocial behavior in children and adolescents*. New York: Oxford University Press.

Kendall, P. C., Furr, J. M., & Podell, J. L. (2010). Child-focused treatment of anxiety. In J. R. Weisz & A. E. Kazdin (Eds.), *Evidence-based psychotherapies for children and adolescents*. New York: Guilford Press.

Koenigsberg, H. W., Harvey, P. D., Mitropoulou, V., Antonia, N. S., Goodman, M., Silverman, J., et al. (2001). Are the interpersonal and identity disturbances in the personality disorder criteria linked to the traits of affective instability and impulsivity? *Journal of Personality, 15*, 358–370.

Kohlenberg, R. J., & Tsai, M. (1993). Functional analytic psychotherapy: A behavioral approach to intensive treatment. In W. O'Donohue & L. Krasner (Eds.), *Theories of behavior therapy: Exploring behavior change*. Washington, DC: American Psychological Association.

Kramer, U., & Zimmerman, G. (2009). Fear and anxiety at the basis of adolescent externalizing and internalizing behaviors. *International Journal of Offender Therapy and Comparative Criminology, 53*, 113–120.

Linehan, M. M. (1993). *Treating borderline personality disorder: The dialectical approach*. New York: Guilford Press.

Linehan, M., Davidson, G., Lynch, T., & Sanderson, C. (2005). Technique factors in treating personality disorders. In L. Castonguay & L. Beutler (Eds.), *Principles of therapeutic change that work*. Oxford University Press.

Links, P. S., Gould, B., & Ratnayake, R. (2003). Assessing suicidal youth with antisocial, borderline, or narcissitic personality disorder. *Canadian Journal of Psychiatry, 48,* 301–310.

Lochman, J. E., & Wells, K. C. (2004). The coping power program for preadolescent aggressive boys and their parents: Outcome effects at one-year follow up. *Journal of Consulting and Clinical Psychology, 72,* 571–578.

Lochman, J. E., Wells, K. C., & Lenhart, L. (2008). *Coping power: Child group facilitators' guide*. New York: Oxford University Press.

McNally, R. J., Malcarne, V. L., & Hansdottir, I. (2001). Vulnerability to anxiety disorders across the lifespan. In R. E. Ingram & J. M. Price (Eds.), *Vulnerability to psychopathology: Risk across the lifespan*. New York: Guilford Press.

Murphy, C. J., & Siv, A. M. (2007). A one year study of mode deactivation therapy: Adolescent residential patients with conduct and personality disorders. *International Journal of Behavioral Consultation and Therapy, 3,* 327–341.

National Institute of Mental Health (n.d.). *Suicide in the U.S.: Statistics and prevention*. Retrieved from http://mentalhealth.gov/health/publications/suicide-in-the-us-statistics-and-prevention/index.shtml#children

O'Brien, K. M., Larson, C. M., & Murrell, A. R. (2008). Third-wave behavior therapies for children and adolescents: Progress and future directions. In L A. Greco & S. C. Hayes (Eds.), *Acceptance and mindfulness treatments for children and adolescents: A practitioner's guide*. Oakland, CA: New Harbinger.

Patterson, G. R. (1982). *Coercive family process*. Eugene, OR: Castalia.

Rohde, P., Clarke, G. N., Mace, D. E., Jorgensen, J., & Seeley, J. R. (2004). An efficacy/ effectiveness study of cognitive-behavioral treatment for adolescents with comorbid major depression and conduct disorder. *Journal of the American Academy of Child and Adolescent Psychiatry, 43,* 660–668.

Stark, K. D., Streusand, W., Krumholz, L. S., & Patel, P. (2010). Cognitive behavioral therapy for depression: The ACTION treatment. In J. R. Weisz, & A. E. Kazdin (Eds.), *Evidence-based psychotherapies for children and adolescents*. New York: Guilford Press.

Tate, D. C., Repucci, N. D., & Mulvey, E. P. (1995). Violent juvenile delinquents: Treatment effectiveness and implications for future action. *American Psychologist, 50,* 777–781.

Weersing, V. R., & Brent, D. A. (2010). Treating depression in adolescents using individual cognitive behavioral therapy. In J. R. Weisz & A. E. Kazdin (Eds.), *Evidence-based psychotherapies for children and adolescents*. New York: Guilford Press.

Weisz, J. R., & Kazdin, A. E. (Eds.). (2010). *Evidence-based psychotherapies for children and adolescents*. New York: Guilford Press.

Wethington, H. R., Hahn, R. A., Fuqua-Whitley, D. S., Sipe, T. A., Crosby, A. E., Johnson, R. L., et al. (2008). The effectiveness of interventions to reduce psychological harm from traumatic events among children and adolescents: A systematic review. *American Journal of Preventive Medicine, 35*, 398–400.

Jack A. Apsche, EdD, ABPP is program director for the masters and doctorate programs in forensic psychology at Walden University and consultant of clinical services at North Spring Behavioral Healthcare. He is founder of the Apsche Center at North Spring in Leesburg, VA. He also serves as editor-in-chief of the *International Journal of Behavioral Consultation and Therapy* and is associate editor of the *Behavior Analyst Today*. He developed, implemented, and tested mode deactivation therapy, which expands on cognitive behavioral therapy and is focused on conceptualizing and treating adolescents. Jack Apsche lives in Leesburg, VA.

Lucia R. DiMeo, PhD, is a licensed clinical psychologist and hypnotherapist. She has a special interest in the research and application of mind/body therapeutic modalities. She is associate professor of psychology at the University of the Virgin Islands. Lucia DiMeo lives in the Caribbean.

Foreword writer **Robert J. Kohlenberg, PhD, ABPP,** is professor of psychology at the University of Washington. He is cocreator of functional analytic psychotherapy (FAP), a behavior analytic approach to understanding the mechanism of action that operates in curative therapist-client relationships.

Index

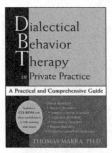
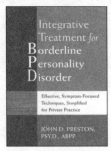
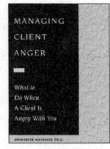
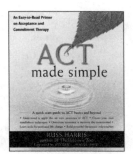
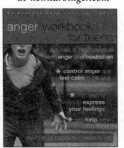
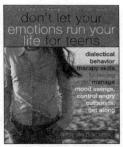
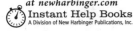
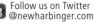
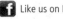

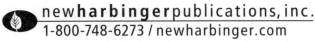